The
METAMORPHIC
Gift

The METAMORPHIC Gift

Simple Techniques to Transform Your Life

Michelle Lindsey-Wehner

DPT, PT, MBA, CPT, Certified KRI Kundalini Yoga
Instructor, and Reiki Practitioner

Printed in the United States

First Printing, 2016

ISBN number 978-0-692-53157-0

Library of Congress Control Number 2015951670

Publisher: Yogacademy
PO Box 44707
Phoenix, Arizona 85064

yogacademybook@gmail.com

Yogacademy.net

Photography: Dr. Robert Lipschultz

Editor: Caryolyn Ruck, Help-U-Write

Cover Design: Ariell Sipel

Interior Design: Caren Cantrell, 102nd Place LLC

Photograph Models: Lindsey Marlais, Michelle Lindsey, Linda Lipschultz

This book is available at quantity discounts for both purchases and for branding by businesses and organizations. For further information or to learn more about Yogacademy, please contact:

Michelle Lindsey-Wehner
PO Box 44707
Phoenix, Arizona 85064

Disclaimer

This book is designed to provide information, education, and inspiration to its readers. It is sold with the understanding that the author and publisher are not engaged in rendering medical, psychological, or other professional advice. **The information contained herein may not be suitable for you. You should consult with a competent professional where appropriate.**

While the author and publisher have used their best efforts in preparing this book, they make no representations or warranties with respect to the accuracy or completeness of the contents and specifically disclaim any implied warranties.

The publisher and the author shall not be liable for any loss or damage either physical, psychological, emotional, legal, financial, commercial or otherwise, including but not limited to special, incidental, consequential, or other damages caused, or alleged to be caused, directly, or indirectly, by the information contained in this book. You are responsible for your choices, actions, and consequences.

You can contact the publisher at www.yogacademy.net about questions or suggestions related to materials, to relay personal experiences in successfully using these or similar techniques, to schedule the author for speaking engagements, or to conduct workshop sessions.

Dedication

This book is dedicated to my son, Cody, who has taught me about listening to my intuition and trusting and having faith in the universe. Cody has shown me the value of living to the fullest and enjoying every precious moment of life. He has also educated me that his giftedness is not a handicap but an asset to society.

The book is also dedicated to all the health professionals who, over the years, have taken my courses and honored and trusted me to help them take a more active role in their own journeys.

Lastly, I cannot forget to thank all my amazing clients who opened their hearts to me, who allowed me to understand the connection between the body and the soul, and who continue to shine a beautiful light of love, protection and confidence around me.

Table of Contents

Acknowledgements

"Develop an attitude of gratitude, and give thanks for everything that happens to you, knowing that every step forward is a step toward achieving something bigger and better than your current situation."
Brian Tracy

As I write these acknowledgements, I look back ten years ago and reflect on the person I was then compared to who I am today. Often, we go through different phases of our life and say to ourselves, "I wish I had done that differently or I wish I had known then what I know now."

I can happily say that I have no regrets or disappointments. Yes, I have had many losses, emotional traumas, physical pains, and days that were difficult for me to get out of bed. These were my personal experiences and I own them, whether they were challenges or gifts. In fact, I firmly believe that all the events leading up today have occurred to help shape my character and to guide me into discovering my soul's purpose in my life.

Uncovering my purpose was similar to finding the missing piece to a puzzle. It was only later in my life that I discovered that my mission was to help improve the overall quality of many peoples' lives by sharing all the information I receive, learn, and experience. I understand that it is through our experiences that we truly gain knowledge. Without my life events, how could I truly put myself in someone else's shoes or really feel compassion and empathy and know the truly deeply rooted pains of life?

My heart is filled with love and gratitude. My appreciation and thanks goes to the universe and to all the universal connections that I have made in my life. I have been provided the insights and shown how to write these words on paper so I could support any person who is struggling to find his/her purpose in life; who wants to understand how the mind-body connects, and who seeks to look within to find valuable tools for self-healing.

It is time to honor yourself, love yourself and discover things about yourself that you have never discovered before. Become aware of your body, mind and spirit, and be grateful to be alive. Allow yourself to release all the "stuff" you have trapped within your body. Detoxify your life and release yourself from fear, judgment, and the past. Breathe in life and fill each breath with love, compassion, happiness, balance, and gratefulness!

Have you noticed how much faster time is moving now and how things are shifting in our world? About eight years ago, I developed a course entitled: *Integrating Neurotherapeutic Techniques and Sensory Techniques into Therapy for the Special Needs Client.* Who knew that all the information I spoke about at that time would be talked about, debated, and now finally become a hot topic?

The funny thing is that after my presentations, I had a lot of health professionals come up to me and ask me if I thought it was my place to talk on that subject and if I was afraid I was opening up a can of worms? And I responded, "Absolutely, it is my place," and I added that all of my information was researched-based. I reported to these individuals that the material I presented needed to be shared. I told them that the material was valuable and well-researched. So, I want to thank those therapists who gave me the opportunity to stand in front of them, allowing me to speak my message. I am grateful because they clarified for me my own conviction that I know what I am speaking about.

I'd like to thank Yogi Bhajan, the man who brought Kundalini Yoga to the Western world in 1969. He is not only deeply missed, but he is also appreciated tremendously for teaching us a set of tools that has helped so many people in their own self-healing to find meaning and purpose in their lives. He is the main inspiration for this book. I feel indebted to him, and I am committed to continue to pass on his teachings to the world, especially the medical world.

I want to thank all my wonderful teachers, healers, and yogic friends who have always given me confirmation that I was walking on the correct path and reminded me to follow my own intuition – that all of the information I needed was all inside of me. They informed me that if I just slowed down and listened, all my answers were waiting to be heard. They helped incorporate new words like "patience, trust, letting go, and having faith" as part of my vocabulary.

I want to thank my amazing, tolerant, giving parents, Linda and Bob Lipschultz, for bringing me into this world and teaching me very strong morals and values. They have kept my light shining because of their love, support, compassion, and guidance in always allowing me to follow my dreams. It wasn't always easy raising a strong willed, sensitive, intuitive woman like me.

I want to thank all the people on my 2009 Yatra and all the people involved in my KRI Level One Immersion course in Espanola, New Mexico. Thank you for creating space for me to grow and evolve and to find balance and stillness within myself.

I want to thank my husband, James Wehner, who has stood by me, protected me, and loved me unconditionally, and has given me one of the biggest blessings of my life, our son CODY.

Lastly, I want to thank my son, Cody, my precious soul, who is a gift to our family and the world. He is a teacher to all. He reminds me every day to love life and be aware of the smallest, most memorable moments in life. His love is contagious to all.

Introduction

My name is Michelle Lindsey. I was born and raised in Northbrook, Illinois. I moved to Phoenix, Arizona, in 1994, where I started a company called Rising Star Therapy Specialists. My company specializes in serving adults and pediatrics with special needs. I am a physical therapist with an eclectic background. But my main desire and passion, not only as the owner of my company but also as a therapist, has been public speaking and creating seminars and books to help spread the word about the latest research that is coming into our field of study.

My previous book, titled *The Wellness Equation: Exploring the Healing Connection between Yoga and Medicine*, is the first book that I wrote as part of a series. This volume, *The Metamorphic Gift,* is a continuation of that series. The knowledge in both books is not only meant for health care professionals, but also for every human being throughout the world. Although some technical terminology is used within this book, the explanations will be simple and understandable so that any ordinary person can easily obtain the information and apply the tools in everyday life.

If you are a health care professional, it would also be most beneficial for you to learn and absorb this material. Why? Because as a health care professional, you are considered a caregiver, and on a daily basis, you are sharing your expertise and wisdom to help clients improve their health status. You, too, have a mission to share what you learn and experience.

I decided to create this book with three reasons or goals in mind. All of them were not only taught to me, but were also shown to me as part of my journey. They came to me from many years of challenges and struggles as I was growing and evolving. They arose throughout my physical therapy career, my athletic background, my worldly travels, my ongoing continuing education, and my responsibilities as a mom and a wife. In other words, they came from all the different roles I played throughout my life and all the years of struggling to find my true self, diminish my ego, and find balance within this high speed, advancing society.

The first purpose or reason is to teach you about **Breath and the Power of the Breath**. The majority of our population does not know how to breathe properly. Do you think that you are breathing correctly? Improper ventilation can lead to medical issues. Wouldn't it be nice to know if you are breathing correctly? In fact, research shows that yogic breathing techniques accelerate therapeutic gains for numerous conditions, such as back pain, scoliosis, tonal issues, temporal mandibular or jaw joint problems, pelvic floor issues, and numerous circulatory and respiratory disorders, not to mention all the calming and refocusing effects it has on the body. It is that simple! Learn to breathe to heal your ailments and prevent future disease.

The second goal is **Body Awareness**. Ask yourself this: "Do you consider your body as an object or something that truly belongs to you?" In other words, do you acknowledge your body or talk to it like an IT? For example, if you have a shoulder problem, do you say, '' My shoulder hurts" or "It hurts?" Giving your problem to someone else and not acknowledging that your shoulder is a part of you will not get you better. Connecting to your body, by looking at your shoulder, talking to it, and touching it with gratitude and love, will definitely make it feel better. Within our society, we prefer someone else to fix our problems. Guess what? You have your own internal tools to connect with your body, and they are free!!

The third reason for designing this book is to teach you how to get out of conformity and into **Creativity.** Do you feel that you are a person who can step out of the box and be creative, or do you feel that you follow what everyone else does? Fear and judgment are often attached with not wanting to step out of the box. As a therapist, I have had the most success when I tune into what my clients need for healing, and then I assist them by creating functional, enjoyable, and out of the ordinary exercises and equipment to help them help themselves. Do I look silly teaching these exercises to my clients? Yes, but they have fun, and I get the honor of discharging them because they feel better.

So, this book is vehicle to expand your information about each of those three important areas, and when you are done reading this book, I guarantee that you will feel more knowledgeable and have all the tools you need to evaluate respiration effectively and create hands on, anytime exercises and body awareness skills. Better yet, you will be able to apply all of this information immediately after you finish the last page of the book. Sound exciting! Are you ready to get started? Let's not wait any longer. Time is ticking!

This book was written so that you will be able to complete the following objectives:

1. Discover how the breath is one of the most important assessment tools in therapeutic evaluation and treatment.
2. Witness how low-back pain can be a result of improper ventilation.

3. Experience how proper ventilation techniques alone can heal a client.
4. Understand how a properly functioning core can keep all of one's anatomical systems balanced.
5. Explore how proper ventilation equates to wellness.
6. Increase your awareness of your body and all your body's connections through education and hands on experience.
7. Recognize ways of exploring and finding your own unique creativity -- of thinking outside the box.

Chapter One: Importance of the Breath

"If there is anything divine in you, it's your breath."
Yogi Bhajan

In this book, you will discover how the power of the breath can help bring overall wellness and vitality to your life. Breath is metamorphic, meaning that when you realize how to breathe correctly and discover how breath affects the entire body, then a complete physical transformation can occur. Your awareness expands, and life becomes clearer and more meaningful. You can understand your Divine purpose in life. Depression, negativity, darkness, anxiety, fear, judgment, ego, pain, emotional turmoil, trauma and drama can all disappear. Your life will become brighter, more beautiful, clearer, creative, light, happy, fun, sensitive, enlightened, pain free, and more empathetic.

Like a caterpillar that was once trapped in a cocoon, you will become free to fly again, seeing the world through a different perspective. Similarly to a butterfly that now has wings to soar, you will have a new vitality in your legs, stepping into hope and aliveness. Just promise that you finish this book in its entirety and I guarantee you will understand how the mind, body, and soul truly connect. Life will make sense and have meaning.

In this book, you will see how Eastern philosophy and Western philosophy intertwine to create a systems model approach to treatment that looks at the body in its entirety and wholeness, without immediately making a judgment or an assumption about what is wrong. You will see that everything is research-based, and that many within clinical practice have had successful outcomes using this book's information. What's more, if you yourself have an ailment or dis-ease, you will learn internal tools to avoid the necessity of always running to the doctor. It is important to sit in your "stuff" and ask yourself with openness, "What it is that I want or desire to become healthy?" Stay in stillness and you will find all the answers within.

The Universe Gets My Attention

Before I began writing Chapter One of this book, I had my own personal experience that I'd like to share. As part of a fertility protocol, for two days my husband had to give me a shot in my buttocks' muscle. According to the doctors, my husband administered the shot in the correct location, but somehow the universe gave me a lesson.

After the shot, I was affected by the most excruciating leg pain that left me in bed for five days, unable to bear my own weight. Throughout the experience, there was electrifying nerve pain throughout my entire leg. In fact, the idea of anyone touching my leg or getting within two inches of my leg created a sympathetic response in my whole body. I felt fear and would begin to sweat, and my heart rate increased. I truly felt debilitated, depressed, and scared. I could relate to my clients who have had this pain which has left them feeling hopeless and depressed.

Normally, my main reaction would have been to reach out for medical help, but instead, I questioned the Universe. First, what was it that I needed to learn from this experience? The answers were readily available. I needed to learn to understand severe, debilitating pain so that I could put myself in the shoes of someone going through this same experience. The second lesson was to recognize that if I could breathe through the pain, I could breathe through the dysfunction.

I was told to imagine a jumper cable connecting my pain-filled leg to my heart and then to breathe deeply, creating a complete circuit and connection between the two. To my surprise, the jumper cable metaphor restarted my body's battery, empowering and circulating energy and blood again. Fortunately, my pain dissipated, and I could walk and smile again. Better yet, my knowledge and wisdom about the power of the breath deepened and became more real.

Lastly, I have to laugh at the other reason why this occurred. The Universe was telling me I needed to stop running around and being busy, so I could sit on my ass, no pun intended, and write this book. It is funny how sometimes lessons can be hard and painful!

The Time for this Approach Is Now

The medical world is changing. How many of you see that today? Throughout society and especially in the business world, there are a lot of shifts taking place financially, socially, and mentally. One of the biggest tools that can benefit us all is to develop our own internal awareness, and that comes from connecting with the breath. A lot of people aren't going to be running to doctors as much as they used to. They're going to have to look within and say, "What is wrong with my body? Can I heal myself?"

I have been a physical therapist for over 20 years now and have had experience in many specialties within my field including orthopedics, wound care, home health, pediatrics, acute care, skilled nursing, and neuro-rehab. My passion today is working with adults and children with special needs. I have traveled all around the United States writing, creating, and speaking on numerous health/wellness related topics such as posture and scoliosis, the connection between yoga and medicine, and sensory integration for the special needs clients. I also hold many certifications in Personal Training, Dry Needling, and Reiki, and I am a Kundalini Research Institute Yoga Teacher.

About seven years ago I desired to write an article in one of our professional magazines on complementary medicine. However, when I reached out to an editor, I was turned down and told that they would not publish any articles on the topic because combining East and West medicine was neither well researched nor commonly used within our profession.

It is wonderful to see how our profession has shifted. A year ago, I was interviewed for the physical therapy magazine, *PT in Motion,* for their July 2014 issue. The article was titled "Integrative Medicine, New Opportunities for PT's." I enjoyed the opportunity explain how I use holistic acupressure and breathing techniques within my practice. The interviewer told me that the term "complementary medicine" was deemed too nonconventional and that the new term coined within our profession was "integrative medicine," and yes, it can be discussed now. A great shift has occurred so that many interventions, once classified as complementary or alternative, are now being integrated into mainstream health care.

Two years ago, I spoke to the American Physical Therapy Association's National Conference on my book, *The Wellness Equation.* I was really excited because I was given the opportunity to step out of the box and speak about the connection between yoga and medicine, a topic at the forefront of our profession. I was extremely honored and blessed to be able to speak on this topic.

After my speaking session, there was a huge gathering of therapists. The guest speaker addressed the future of our profession. A new vision statement was created: *Transforming society by optimizing movement to improve the human experience.* Physical therapists are encouraged to step out of the box and be more creative in our thinking process.

I felt deeply inspired as we were guided to understand and use the terms wellness and prevention within our vocabulary. We were encouraged to incorporate new tools into our practice such as Yoga, Pilates and Dry Needling – tools from Eastern Medicine Philosophy.

My personal belief was that it was time to welcome these new tools because as medical professionals, we must grow with our profession.

Furthermore, the speaker emphasized that clinical research will always lag behind clinical practice. How many of you are always questioning, "Is that research-based? Are we allowed to do that technique if it's not research-based?" Perhaps we need to shift our focus and certainly remember that experience gained through clinical practice is also important.

Moving Into the New Paradigm

I'd like to share with you my thoughts on the new vision or paradigm mentioned above: *Transforming society by optimizing movement to improve the human experience.* As physical therapists, we study movement. Movement, to me, not only involves the activation of our muscles but also the act or process of moving people or things from one idea to another. This movement involves awareness and making choices for a more successful and healthy existence.

I feel that the current shift within our profession to use the systems model approach encompasses this new paradigm. The systems model approach makes us, as physical therapists, look deeper into the cause of a client's problem or illness before immediately making an assumption or judgment. This simply means looking at the whole client and not just the illness. Thus, it involves looking at the human body in its complete wellness-multidimensionality: physically, mentally, spiritually, socially, occupationally, and environmentally.

It is important that, as therapists, we must meet our clients' needs and help them to maintain a more balanced state of health along all sectors. As therapists, we must move and change our health practices so we can aid our clients to make healthy lifestyle changes. Using this new paradigm then requires a new set of tools in our thinking.

For example, there is research that our higher cognitive processes – our minds – are grounded in our body experiences and in the neural circuitry that controls our body. Therefore, all of the information we gather from our world comes through our senses. Integrative medicine uses our own body's circuitry to send messages and information for self-healing. The idea is that the client needs to understand how to connect to his or her body. They need to become aware!

Therefore, as physical therapists, we need to gain skills in integrative medicine. These tools include the following – the PT must be able to:

- observe and interpret what the client is not saying or is saying;
- train the client to think differently about his or her illness;
- show the client how to use his or her hands to create bodily changes instead of always having the PT do the manual, hands-on work;
- gain better listening skills and avoid relying on the PT's ego to immediately think in a certain programmed way;
- teach a client how to breathe correctly and to use the breath with movement;
- train the client to see the world through his or her true perspective.

This direction of change within our profession will help the client can gain better bodily movement and be able to advance to optimal health.

Think About Managing Your Health as You Would Manage Your Finances

Yogi Bhajan, who brought Kundalini Yoga to the Western world said, "The Ocean is a very calm thing. But when the winds are heavy and high, then it's choppy. The wind represents your ego, and the higher the ego, the choppier is a person's life."

To understand this quote a little better, my friend – a teacher and financial advisor – told me a story about one of her classes. She was teaching the students about finance and she asked them, "Does anyone have a dollar bill?" All the students raised their hands. The teacher pointed to a young lady and said, "I want your dollar bill." The student then gave the teacher the dollar bill. The teacher looked at the class, took out a lighter, and burned the dollar bill right in front of all the students.

All the students questioned, "What is she doing?" The instructor looked at them and said, "I am going to teach you all a valuable lesson today. I want you to learn how to manage your own money. I want you to learn how to rely on no one else but yourself, because in this world, some people are always going to take advantage of you. They're going to want to take your money. Because of their own egos, they're going to want to do things with your money in ways that you may not agree with. They may say that they're going to make you lot of money, but the point is that I want to teach you about your own finances."

In the same way that teacher told her students that she wanted them to be knowledgeable about their own finances, I want to teach you about your own breath. I want to teach you about your own body awareness. I want you to complete this book and say, "NOW, I have the internal tools to know what's actually going on in my body".

Chapter Two: The Power of the Breath

"If you want to conquer the anxiety of life, live in the moment, live in the breath."
Amit Ray

The Power of Breath

Let's begin by speaking about the breath. The breath is considered prana, our life force. Think about it for a moment. Without breath, there is no life. We need the breath to keep us alive.

Henry David Thoreau once said, "We are all sculptors and painters and our material is our own flesh and blood and bones."Our breath is crucial to our mind, our body, and our hygiene.

The breath supplies our body with the most vital nutrient that we need for survival. And what's that most vital nutrient? It's oxygen. We can survive without food for weeks and water for days, but without oxygen, we will die within minutes. (Bagus, J, 2013).

We need to enrich our body with oxygen and get rid of all the toxins in our system. These toxins may have accumulated from years of bad habits, addiction issues, or poor posture. In order to circulate oxygen and eliminate toxins, we must learn how to breathe properly.

The organ within our body that needs the most oxygen is our brain. The brain is responsible for our vision, our hearing, our mobility, our emotions, our positive and negative thoughts, our memory and speech, and a bunch of other functions. If the brain isn't getting enough oxygen, then the other organs of our body will not survive.

At a deeper level, Jennifer Bagus, in her article titled "The Importance of Breathing," describes the breath as the one special fiber that unites an individual to the universe. She reminds us that we are all connected through the breath. Breath is also a reminder of the gift of life – that every moment is precious. Most of us today are so busy with life that we walk around stressed and don't fully expand our lungs. By taking the time to connect with our breath, we can truly experience what life is all about.

In the Orient, there is a saying that when a child is born, the lifespan is already predetermined or preset, not by the number of years but by the number of breaths allotted. (Bagus, J, 2013) So, by breathing slowly, you will live longer. You'll live a healthier, lengthier life.

As humans, we have a lifespan of about 100 years. Proper ventilation, with a slower rate of breathing, can impact everything – a stronger nervous system, a healthier lymphatic system, improved circulation, enhanced respiration, and overall better immunity.

Bonnie Bainbridge Cohen is an Occupational Therapist and the developer of Body-Mind Centering. She wrote, "Breathing is automatic. It is influenced by internal physiological and psychological states and by external environmental factors . . . The way we breathe will also influence our behavior and our physical functioning".

She also said, "Breathing is an internal movement. It underlies the movement of body through external space. So movement in turn, will alter our breathing . . . Breathing is organized in patterns. And these patterns are influenced by our emotional stimuli. They also evoke emotional responses . . . Our first breath at birth, very importantly, will influence our pattern of adult breathing, and that breathing can be consciously known." As the breathing process is sensed and felt, unconscious blocks can be released.

When you become aware of your breath, you may start to feel really connected. So breathing is not only physical. It's emotional. It brings vitality, and it brings this consciousness or connection to everyone and to the universe. (Cohen, B., 2012).

Who are the best breathers? Babies. Why? Because babies know how to breathe in and out of their nose and they know how to activate their diaphragms. When we are born, we are born as nasal breathers. We don't have the voluntary ability to actually breathe out of our mouth. Realize that mouth breathing is a learned response that is activated by some emergency situation. For example, if an infant's nose becomes blocked, suddenly, they'll start to suffocate or cry. And what will they do? The crying forces air into their mouth and lungs. Mouth breathing allows large volumes of air into their lungs for survival so the baby can return to nasal breathing (Engles, L, 2006).

Make some time to observe a baby sleeping. I loved the nights when I would sit up watching our son breathe. It was meditative and peaceful. It is no surprise that all the research today states that all the cerebral spinal fluid, which is a clear, colorless liquid that cleans the brain and spinal cord, is balanced by secretion through the nasal sinuses. Blocking this self-bathing mechanism is connected to a large portion of our headaches and other medical issues (Bhajan, Yogi, 2007).

Each nostril, as you will understand more fully later on in this book, is innervated or stimulated by five different cranial nerves from each side of the brain. Each nostril functions independently and synergistically, helping to filter, warm, moisturize, dehumidify and smell the air. The nasal sinuses balance the pH. They also decrease water loss, helping with hydration, and aid in slowing the air escape so the lungs have more time to extract oxygen from them.

Moreover, afferent nerve fibers that carry stimuli to the brain to regulate breathing are located in the nasal passages. Did you know that nasal breathing stimulates the parasympathetic nervous system, the part of the autonomic nervous system that is responsible for rest and digestion? The parasympathetic system calms the mind and helps the body. In contrast, mouth breathing causes a fight or flight response causing the release of cortisol and adrenaline, leading to more rapid aging, cancer, disease, and death. Mouth breathing even causes fat storage.

There even is a correlation between nasal breathing and heart rate. The diaphragm will become stronger with nasal breathing, supplying the body with longer, deeper breaths. The average athlete who uses mouth breathing breathes 30-40 breaths per minute during exercise. With nasal breathing, the number of breaths is halved. This equates to increased performance (Engles, L, 2006, and Optimal 2 Breathing Mastery, 2014). It you learn how to breathe correctly, chant, or hum, you can even clear your sinuses and stop nasal congestion (Bond, M, 2007).

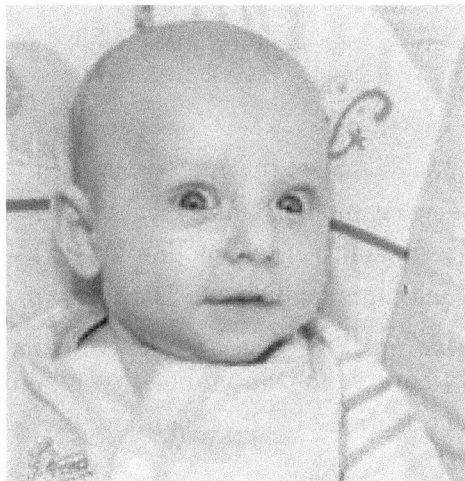

Now You Try It

Let's take a moment and experience the difference between mouth breathing and nasal breathing. My goal is to have you actually connect with your body.

Sit back in a comfortable chair with your spine straight and head in neutral. It is time to go within and sit with your breath.

Close your eyes. I want you to take a moment and just breathe in and out of your mouth. Notice if the breath stays in your chest or does it move towards your diaphragm around the navel area? Are you breathing through your chest or diaphragm?

Keep your eyes closed, close your mouth, and breathe in and out of your nose. Now where does the breath go? Is it in your chest or your diaphragm around the navel area?

The answer: mouth-breathing keeps the breath more in the upper chest and neck area, whereas nose breathing activates the diaphragm, navel area, the chest, and neck area. People who hyperventilate are usually mouth-breathing. Someone who is hyperventilating should be immediately told to breathe in and out of their nose.

Mouth Breathing Versus Nose Breathing

Why have we become mouth breathers? One of the main reasons is because of our habits and how we take care of our bodies. Over time, our habits can become more pronounced. In fact, it is difficult, or at least challenging, to stay a nose-breather within our society today. Everything seems faster paced. When we are in a hurry or stressed out, our breathing patterns change. Geographical location, age, posture, trauma, anxiety, the media, and even our self-esteem play a part in how we breathe.

Most importantly, it is our first breath that is the most important breath. Remember, the moment that you are severed from your mother's umbilical cord is the first time that your circulatory system and respiratory system has to function on its own. The lungs have to operate for the first time. Additionally, the baby has to learn how to suck and swallow. He or she is no longer weightless in a fluid filled environment. Babies have to learn how to be supported by gravity and not only have stabilization, but also mobilization. Their muscles have to evolve to help with posture, learning balance and how to support the weight of the head (Kandoff, L, 2007).

Yogi Bhajan used to say that babies actually do 108 postures within the womb. It is not surprising then that when babies enter the world, they are the most flexible beings. Have you ever just watched babies move? I personally am amazed. I can't imagine my body doing some of those postures. Because of this amazing flexibility, the body naturally becomes open to receiving more oxygen. All the bodies' connections, especially the diaphragm's connections, are neither restricted nor inhibited.

Furthermore, from birth to six weeks, you'll see babies breathing about 30 to 60 breaths per minute. At three years old, babies breathe about 20 to 30 breaths per minute. Adults usually will breathe 12 to 20 breaths per minute. Men actually breathe about 16 to 18 breaths per minute, whereas women breathe a little bit slower than men, 18 to 20 breaths per minute. The reason why babies breathe more rapidly is because the baby's thorax and lungs are the same size, and the lungs are not stretched out yet to fit the relaxed rib cage. Therefore, infants must breathe two to three times as often as an adult with adequate respiration. In adults, the lungs fit the rib cage and as a result, adults have a greater increased capacity and reserve than infants (Anatomy and Physiology for Speech, Language, and Hearing, 2010). The above rates are normal, but when babies grow and develop, their breathing rate will become more like adults. As you will see, you will learn how to lower your own breathing rates through various breathing exercises.

The benefits of proper breathing are the release stress and tension, so relaxed breathing equates to diaphragmatic breathing. Gary Hendricks wrote a book called *Conscious Breathing* in 1995. He summarizes that proper breathing builds energy and endurance, contributes to emotional mastery, prevents and heals physical problems, contributes to graceful aging, and helps manage pain. The breath can even aid in improving mental concentration and physical performance. Gary Hendricks also stated that breathing is the path to the most essential of human experience leading to love.

As far as disease prevention is concerned, the breath can help with problems like asthma, bronchitis, COPD, emphysema, anxiety, panic attacks, sports performance, blood pressure reduction, headaches and migraines, sleep problems, smoking cessation, stress management and weight loss. It can even relieve Paradoxical Vocal Cord Dysfunction which is when the vocal cords close when they should open during the respiratory cycle. It is often mistaken for asthma.

The mind is a huge component in how we breathe. The two must work together as a team. The rate of your breath must be balanced by your state of mind. The breath can help guide the mind and then the body follows. With a slower rate of breathing, you can have better control over your mind (Bagus, J, 2013 and Khalsa, S.P.K, 1996).

Tests are available to assess how well your lungs work by measuring how much air you inhale, how much you exhale, and how fast you exhale. The results from these tests can be used to diagnose pulmonary diseases like asthma, COPD, and emphysema.

Many respiratory diseases affect the organs and tissues that make gas exchange possible. The most common obstructive airway diseases are asthma, COPD, and Cystic Fibrosis. Asthma is a condition where airways are continuously inflamed, causing bronchial spasms, wheezing, and shortness of breath. It is usually triggered by pollution and infections. COPD is an inability to exhale normally causing difficulty breathing. Cystic Fibrosis is a genetic condition causing poor clearance of mucus from the bronchi, causing airways to become reduced in volume or have free flow of gas hindered, creating a challenge for air to move in and out of the lungs. The demarcation point for airway obstruction is the point at which less than 70 percent of the vital capacity can be expired in one second. (Vemier, 2014)

Restrictive lung diseases, on the other hand, result in a loss of lung compliance, leading to diminished lung expansion and amplified lung stiffness. Examples of restrictive lung diseases are obesity, scoliosis, and neuromuscular diseases like muscular dystrophy or amyotrophic lateral sclerosis (ALS).

A way to obtain respiratory measurements is by using a spirometer. Spirometry looks at volume changes that happen in a closed circuit and that are measured while an individual is breathing through a mouthpiece into a measures device. (Vemier, 2014 and Lung Disease and Respiratory Health Center)

One measurement that can be assessed is vital capacity or the amount of air that can be forcefully exhaled following a maximum inspiration. Inspiration is defined as drawing in of the breath, whereas expiration is breathing out or forcing air out of the lungs. Research with athletes has found no difference in the average vital capacities of pre-pubescent and Olympic wrestlers and trained middle distance athletes compared with untrained healthy athletes, showing us that it is genetic endowment and strengthened muscles due to specific exercise training that is responsible for performance (Mc Ardle, D, Katch, F.and D, 1991).

Another important measurement is called total lung capacity. Total lung capacity is defined as the maximum amount of air in the lungs at the end of a maximum inspiration. One component involved in the measurement of total lung capacity is residual volume, which is the amount of air remaining in the lungs after maximum expiration. This is the amount of air that can never be voluntarily exhaled. The actual lung volume or capacity is 6000 ml (milliliters) which is equivalent to 6000 cc. (cubic centimeters). So, imagine that you are blowing up a balloon, and the balloon represents your total lung capacity. If you are using 6000 cc of air, you will fully fill up this balloon. However, if you are unable to use your total lung capacity for various reasons then imagine that you are only filling only 1/10th of the balloon up with air.

Don't worry so much about the number, but understand that you and I may only be using 600 to 700 cubic centimeters of air with each breath we take. It is important to remember that we need full lung expansion to not only properly clean the mucous lining in the small air sacs of the lungs but also to get rid of toxic irritants in them.

I'll bet you are wondering why this number is so small? Most people breathe from their chest, and they don't properly activate the diaphragm or navel center. When I speak of the movement of the breath, I'm going to talk about it in three parts. The flow of the breath should occur first from the abdominal area, then to the chest area (upper and lower), and finally to the neck area to include the jaw and clavicular area.

Imagine your breath is climbing from the pelvic region all the way to the head and neck area. Mouth breathing works the chest area, but diaphragmatic breathing works all three of these steps. Guess what? If the diaphragm isn't functioning properly, then there will be little energy or oxygen flow to the pelvis, lower extremities, the back, and even to the jaw. Can you see how restricted breathing can lead to many disorders?

To summarize, one of my goals in writing this book is to try and help you lower the number of your breaths per minute in order to help get more oxygen and blood flow to the system. This activity can be accomplished by exploring the direct relationship between gravity, posture, and the breath.

Insights from My Own Experience

In my twenties, I was an elite marathon runner who had many medical issues. These problems ranged from kidney stones to thyroid problems to digestive issues. The only thing that was healthy was my ego.

After many years of medications and suffering, I left the United States with an amazing bunch of people to study yoga and meditation in India. I found myself in this energetic country and did not want to leave.

As I took training to be a yoga teacher and a big advocate of the breath, I discovered that all along I was breathing incorrectly. I was a paradoxical breather, meaning that I really never activated my diaphragm area, but used my chest area instead. With paradoxical breathing, my chest wall would move in on inspiration and on expiration it would move out. This is opposite of how the breath really works. My stomach was sucked in tightly, continuously depriving me of oxygen and proper diaphragmatic breathing. So, I was not circulating blood and oxygen very well throughout my body, leading to the above medical problems.

As soon as I learned the functional anatomy of how the breath works and understood it, I was able to heal myself, lessen my medications, and minimize my doctors' visits. I was able to apply the knowledge I learned from my own personal experience to my clients. I began assessing them and I soon discovered that the majority of them did not know how to breathe properly. Sure enough, once my clients learned how to breathe correctly and apply this understanding to their exercise programs and to their lives, they did not need to return to my practice. They were healed, and I was truly grateful that they had discovered the power of the breath.

Dysfunctional Breathing and Asthma

Did you know that people with dysfunctional breathing are often misdiagnosed as having asthma? Hagman, Janson, and Emtner in 2008 did a study titled *"A Comparison between Patients with Dysfunctional Breathing and Patients with Asthma."* Over a five year span, they focused on breathing retraining for patients with dysfunctional breathing. With proper diaphragmatic training, patients with dysfunctional breathing were less impaired by their breathing problems both in daily life and exercising. Their quality of live improved, physical symptoms lessened, and the number of emergency room visits declined. The symptoms of dysfunctional breathing also decreased.

There is a test for people 12 years and older called the ACT or Asthma Control Test. It is simply a five question health survey used to measure asthma control. The Nijmegen Questionnaire is also available to take as well. It gives a broad view of symptoms associated with dysfunctional breathing patterns. This questionnaire will tell a client if he/she has problems with over breathing or hyperventilation.

Proper breathing involves the diaphragm. The diaphragm is a major player of breath, responsible for about 70 to 80 percent of our breathing. It separates the thoracic cavity from the abdominal cavity. It is a dome-shaped sheet of muscle that is approximately 1/8 of an inch thick. It creates the roof of the abdomen and the floor of the rib cage.

The outside of the diaphragm attaches all the way around the lower border of the ribs, from the spine in the rear to the breastbone on the front. Its domed top lies about halfway between the lower front ribs and the nipple line. The diaphragm is attached to the pleura, connective tissue surrounding the lungs. The motion of the diaphragm contracts and flattens the dome of the abdomen which pulls on the lungs. In respiration, the diaphragm contract during inhalation and enlarges the thoracic cavity. It relaxes and air is exhaled during exhalation.

The heart and lungs rest above the diaphragm, while the liver, stomach, gallbladder, pancreas, bladder, and intestines sit below it. The diaphragm is innervated by the phrenic nerve which runs through the cervical vertebrae and connects the C3, C4, and C5 vertebrae. There is a saying I learned in physical therapy school, "C3, C4, C5, keeps the diaphragm alive".

If you have a client with a cervical spine or neck issue, wouldn't it be wise to first evaluate if they are breathing correctly? How many physical therapists evaluate the breath upon observation for any illness? I will soon show you how important this valuable tool, the breath, is for evaluation and treatment.

The diaphragm also has a role in non-respiratory functions, such as vomiting, feces, expelling urine from the body by increasing pressure within the abdomen, and preventing acid reflux. The diaphragm has three openings, one for the inferior vena cava at T8; T10 for the esophagus; and T12 for the aorta.

Breathing

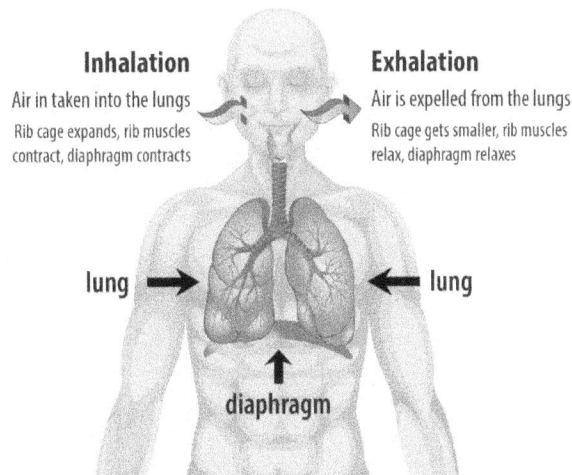

Inhalation
Air in taken into the lungs
Rib cage expands, rib muscles
contract, diaphragm contracts

Exhalation
Air is expelled from the lungs
Rib cage gets smaller, rib muscles
relax, diaphragm relaxes

lung

lung

diaphragm

Breathing and Acid Reflux: Cody's Experiences

Have you ever suffered from heart burn? I'd like to tell you a story about my son that illustrates the connection between the diaphragm and the esophagus.

After my son was born, he cried for six months. Every woman who has a baby wants the perfect child who sleeps, has a good temperament and is calm. This was not my case. When I gave birth to my son, Cody came out crying. He cried for twenty four hours a day and had to be held all the time because it was too painful for him to lie on his back.

I was literally in a torture chamber with a crying baby and little support. During that first six months, I lost all my pre-pregnancy weight plus more. I cried with my son because I felt hopeless. I went to three pediatricians who advised me that my son was colicky. To me the term "colicky" is just a diagnosis telling me that the doctors had no idea what was wrong with him.

As a physical therapist, I firmly believe that there is always a cause for a problem but some digging deep is required to find a solution. So I felt that I personally had to find a solution if the doctors' were unable to do so.

Cody's symptoms included keeping his body in flexed posturing. He would turn bright red as if he was in pain He was unable to be flat on his back and he wanted unstoppable breast feeding all day long. The one symptom that helped me figure out what was wrong was that he constantly arched his back for pressure relief. This unusual movement pattern sent me searching for the right pediatrician.

Finally, with prayer, I found a pediatrician that could help me. When I met her, I cried in her office and begged her to help me. She diagnosed my son with acid reflux. The pediatrician explained to me that Cody's diaphragm wasn't fully developed and his rib cage was tight and pushing on his diaphragm. And since the diaphragm has a hole for the esophagus at T10, what was happening was that Cody's diaphragm was compressing on his esophagus, pushing all the acid up his throat. His throat was literally burning when he was lying flat because the acid was moving up to his throat. Arching his back allowed his diaphragm to expand and open up so that the acid wouldn't go up to his throat anymore.

Think about it. When you swallow, your food must pass down a long tube known as the esophagus into your stomach. This tube must pass through the diaphragm. The opening in the diaphragm is regulated by a sphincter muscle which opens when we swallow food to allow it to pass through the diaphragm and into the stomach. This sphincter also shuts to prevent acid from coming up to the throat.

In many cases, a hiatal hernia can occur because the top of the stomach moves up into the opening and becomes wedged. If a hiatal hernia results, it can look like other diseases. Why? The tight position of the stomach can stress the vagus nerve which fuels the release of hydrochloric acid, causing both, too little, or too much release of stomach enzymes or hydrochloric acid.

Irritation on this nerve can also cause irritations in the body since the vagus nerve comes from the medulla, part of the brain, and moves to the heart, esophagus, lungs, stomach, small intestine, liver, gallbladder, pancreas, and colon. The movement of the diaphragm can also become affected. The esophagus can twist in the throat, causing problems with swallowing and thyroid gland issues, similar to my son's case (Wilder, Bee, 2013).

Fortunately, my son's acid reflux was not the result of a hiatal hernia. With proper positioning, loosening up his diaphragm and rib cage area, craniosacral and chiropractic work, and medication, Cody's acid reflux diminished

Remember, that if a client has a tight rib cage or a weak diaphragm or other diaphragmatic issues, this can affect his or her entire system, including the client's energetic body. Looking a little bit outside the box for a solution to a problem can prove very beneficial, as I discovered.

Finding Your Navel Center

In my practice of Kundalini yoga, the focus of the breath is on the navel center. In my physical therapy practice, this area is equivalent to what is called the Core.

The navel area is an energetic center or a center of energy transformation in the body. It can help move energy throughout the body, from the bottom of the feet to the top of the head. It helps in the connection between the diaphragm, the pelvic floor, the back, the neck, and the brain.

This navel center is considered the major focus of all movement. When any exercise or yogic posture is performed, focus is on movement around this center. It is located a few inches below the navel, in front of the spine.

Place your index finger on your belly button. Now place your middle and ring fingers of the same hand directly next to your index finger. Make sure that all three fingers are on your body. Now lift up the index finger and the middle finger, and where your ring finger is lying is where the energy center of your system will be.

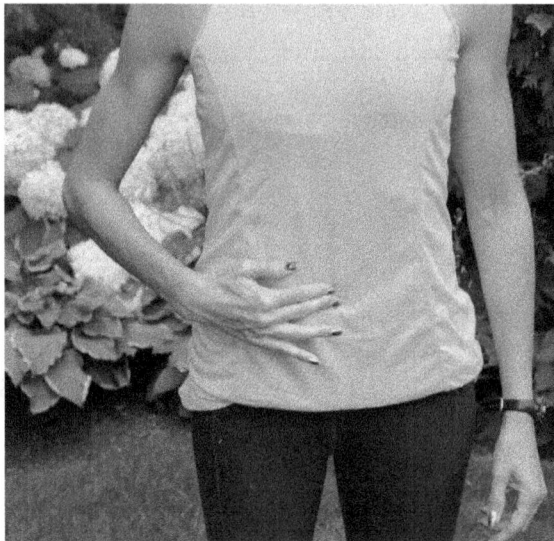

The Naval Point

This is your core energetic center. Imagine that a pole is going directly though this center. You are only allowed to move through this center. Therefore, if you are moving forward, backward, bending, or reaching, you must keep this energy center open by moving in and around it. When this center is open, the breath will move as it should. Your connective tissue connections within your body will be unrestricted and you will feel more balanced and alive.

In men, this navel center displaces to the left and in females it displaces to the right. It has its own beat. If the navel beat is found above the belly button, constipation, improper digestion, acidity and diseases of the heart can occur. If it is displaced downwards, colic pain and loose stools can occur. Moreover, if displaced sideways, acute pain can result. In females, displacement can lead to menstrual irregularities (Bhajan, Yogi, 2007).

Proper Movement Affects Breathing

Take a moment and reach for something across a table. Then reach for something on the floor. I'll bet that you bent from the waist and did not move from your energetic center. If you bent from the waist, it is most likely that your head bent forward, followed by your shoulders. Just by doing this movement you have compressed your diaphragm, shut off your pelvic floor, and limited the usage of your back muscles. Continuous, habitual patterns like this will lead to further medical issues. Your awareness of the quality of your movement is essential for wellness and overall health.

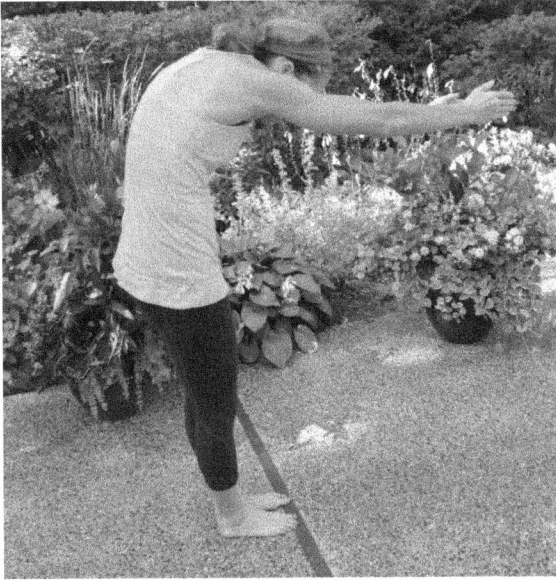

Improper Reaching

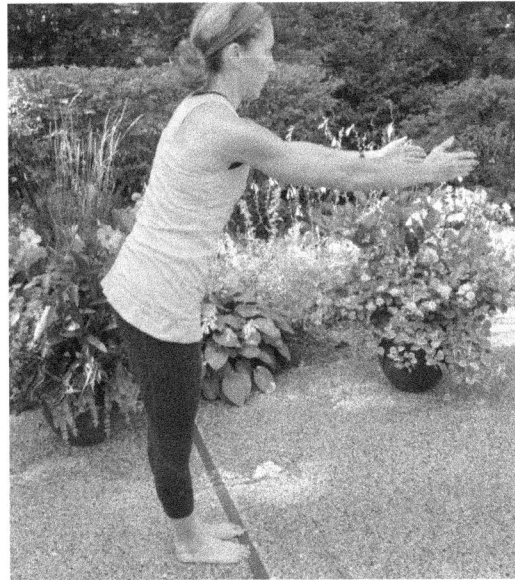

Proper Reaching

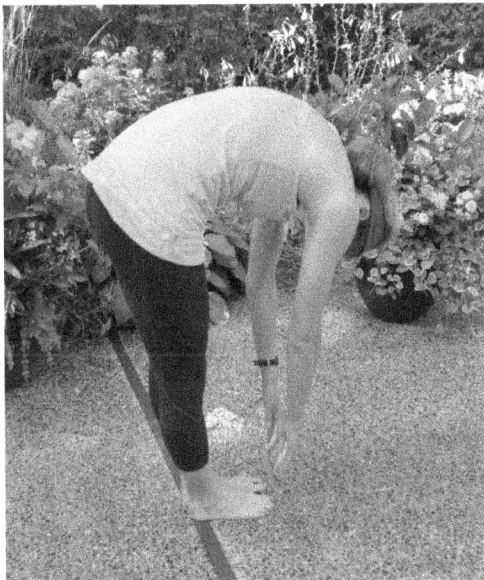

Improper Bending

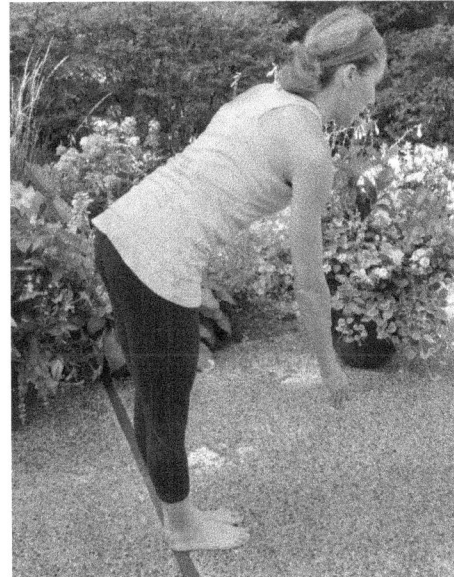

Proper Bending

So How Do You Know If You're Breathing Correctly

Knowing all this, let's see if you are breathing correctly and can begin to experience how it feels to be within your body. Close your eyes and sit in a supported chair with your spine and head in neutral and gently place both your hands on your navel center.

Now go within and focus on your breathing. Inhale and exhale and feel the breath move within your body. If upon inspiration, your navel center is moving in and on exhalation your navel center is moving out, you are doing paradoxical or backwards breathing. It is important to realize this and know that with practice you can breathe correctly.

Let's talk about the diaphragm. The diaphragm is a major pump. Think about how a pump can go up and down all the time. The diaphragm is your pump, and proper breathing involves the proper movement of this pump.

Upon inhalation, this muscle or pump will move downward toward the navel center. When the diaphragm moves down it pulls on the pleura of the lungs. The lungs open up and expand like a balloon. The lungs look for vital nutrients and oxygen to fill up their space. At the same time, the navel center expands too, meaning your abdominal area moves out. Your body becomes like a balloon, receiving and absorbing oxygen from all angles of the environment.

The breath can now fill up the three steps mentioned earlier: the abdominal area, the lower and upper chest area, and the head, neck, and jaw area. If the breath can't circulate to the jaw area, it can cause headaches, temporal mandibular or jaw issues, and neck problems.

The breath needs to circulate all over the body with inhalation so all anatomical systems can work together. These systems include the respiratory system, circulatory system, lymphatic system, digestive system, musculoskeletal system, the reproductive system, the nervous system, and the endocrine system. What's more, when inhalation is working correctly, the spine can extend.

The diaphragm has a connective tissue connection to the deep back muscles, the lumbar multifidi. If you are a paradoxical breather, the spine will not extend. The deep back muscles will not be innervated much, leading to low back problems. Also, you will not be circulating blood flow and oxygen very well, almost like reversing your blood flow.

To summarize, when you inhale, the diaphragm drops, the navel center goes out, air fills your entire body, and the spine extends. With exhalation, the opposite occurs: the diaphragm pushes up, inflating the lungs and removing all toxins and carbon monoxide out to the environment. The navel center moves in or moves towards the spine, and the spine moves back to neutral. With exhalation, you will say goodbye to oxygen, toxins, and nutrients that do not serve your body anymore. Breathing, inhaling and exhaling correctly, is like giving your body a full body massage.

Now take a moment and focus on your breath. Are you breathing correctly now? It is important to learn how to breathe correctly so we can use the breath with exercise. Conscious breathing involves being aware of your breath and connecting with your breath at a deeper, mind, body, and spirit level. Your goal by the end of the book is to breathe every breath with awareness and consciousness. Don't forget to breathe in and out through your nose.

Chapter Three: The Role of Connective Tissue

"A typical neuron makes about ten thousand connections to neighboring neurons. This means there as many connections in a single cubic centimeter of brain tissue as there are stars in the Milky Way galaxy."
David Eagleman

What is connective tissue? Connective tissue is a term for all the tissues of the body that separate, contain, and connect everything else within the body. Connective tissue is made of a viscous matrix called "ground substance" that is either more fluid or more solid depending on the demands placed on it. It is similar in texture to a thick lubricating gel.

Connective tissue has different names depending on its location and function.
Ligaments are the fibrous connective tissue that attach bone to bone.
Tendons secure muscle to bone.

Bone is a highly mineralized form of connective tissue. The covering around our nerves and blood vessels is also made of connective tissue. Most importantly, the sheaths around our organs and muscles are made up of connective tissue called Fascia.

Our bodies contain a three dimensional web of fascia with pockets and tubes around many of our organs and muscles and around compartments of every cell. Fascia is a band or sheet of connective tissue that is like the glue that binds everything together. It is the support network of the body.

Think of fascia as having properties similar to a sweater. The web of fibers of the sweater goes in all different directions similar to fascia within the body. If you get a snag in the sweater, the support structure of the sweater will not fit the same on you. It may pull more on one shoulder than the other, creating imbalance. This imbalance couples with other forces throughout the sweater, throwing the whole sweater out of alignment (The Caroline Theme, 2014).

Connective tissue or fascia is made up of three components. Elastin fibers are similar to rubber bands that stretch and recoil. Collagen is composed of long tough threads that provide support. The more tightly these threads are woven, the stronger this part of the fascia is. The ground substance is the lubricating gel that provides shock absorption. Thus, fascia is strong, pliable and flexible and can withstand impact (Pearlscott, M, 1999-2015).

Connective tissue makes up 20% of one's body weight (Bond, 2007). Connective tissue provides a communication network that is different from other modes of communicating within our bodies. The "ground substance" of connective tissue has a liquid crystalline structure and it conducts bioelectric energy. With compression and stretching, these currents create changes in the fascia state.

Fascia stabilizes your posture. If a person has poor posture, this signaling of the currents causes the fascia to produce more fiber which results in chronic issues. Fascia shrinks and toughens in response to any kind of stress or muscle tightness. Because the fascia connects all body regions, adhesion in one place can create strain in distant areas. For example, a tight knee can cause adhesions around digestive organs or an imbalanced head position may be due to hearing loss (Bond, M. 2007).

The Importance of Core Stabilization

Throughout the ages, the movement that brings the navel towards the spine has been known as "core" stabilization and is recognized as an essential concept of good coordination and health. Current understanding is that this movement involves a co-contraction of lumbar multifidus and of transversus abdominis, specifically the sub-umbilical portion (Newton, A., 1995, 1997, 2004). The transversus abdominus and lumbar multifidus do not move the spine, but stabilize it so that the other muscles can move the trunk without compromising the integrity of the joints.

Think of the lumbar multifidus as a line of deep muscle along your spine. The muscular line originates at the neck and extends all the way to the base of the spine. It helps stabilize your spine, and back injuries can involve this deep muscle.

The transversus abdominus is like a muscle girdle that stabilizes the pelvis. Like a girdle, when this muscle is activated, it will help thin the waist and flatten your stomach. Drawing in this area of the belly to flatten the back is key in all the movements of Tai Chi, Pilates and Yoga.

The lumbar multifidi and transversus abdominus are examples of local muscles, while rectus abdominus and the external obliques are examples of global muscles. The rectus abdominus or "washboard" is the abdominal muscle familiar to most people. It runs vertically from the pelvis to the 5-7 ribs and to the tip of the sternum. The external obliques can be visualized as the superficial muscles on the lateral sides of the abdominal region. These muscles work when you are side bending or doing a side plank.

Engagement of the rectus abdominus while exercising is likely to pull the chest and pelvis together, compressing the diaphragm. Wanting to have a "six pack" or "a ripped abdominal area" may get you in trouble. Additionally, sit-ups and lumbar extension exercises most often do not differentiate between global and local muscle involvement and may not be the answer to solving low back pain.

Along with the transversus abdominus and lumbar multifidi, the diaphragm and the pelvic floor are often included in the structures involved in core stabilization. Preliminary studies have revealed that when a limb is moved, the contraction of the pubococcygeus (a part of the pelvic floor) occurs concurrently with that of the transversus abdominis. Carolyn Richardson and her colleagues in Australia investigated the role of these muscles in back pain with healthy patients. In Richardson's experiment, the researchers found that only 10% of those with a history of low back pain could activate the transversus abdominis compared with 82% of the non-low-back-pain subjects. They found that patients who performed exercises that specifically targeted the transversus abdominis over the course of 10 weeks experienced a significant decrease in pain and an increase in functional ability compared to the control group which received conventional treatments such as swimming, workouts and sit-ups (Newton, A.C, 1995, 1997, 2004).

Additionally, in some research studies, patients with chronic low back pain appear to have both abnormal position and a steeper slope of the diaphragm when using isometric flexion against resistance of the upper and lower extremities was applied (Kolar, KP, Sulc J., Kynel M., Sanda J., Cakt O., Andel R., Kumagai K., Kobesova A., 2012). Another study showed that the multifidus and the other muscles along the spine are significantly smaller in patients with chronic low back pain, especially on the side where symptoms of chronic low back pain occur as compared with the asymptomatic side. There was also a decrease in the mass of the multifidus muscle at the fourth and fifth lumbar vertebrae as compared to the control patients who are healthy. (Fortin, M., Macedo, L., 2013)

All the diaphragms of the body -- respiratory and pelvic as well as the palate, and even the feet and hands -- can be seen as part of a single functional system. The answer to having a strong core is having a healthy, functioning diaphragm and that is obtained through correct breathing.

Getting Acquainted with Your Own Body

Before I move on, I'd like to familiarize you with your transversus abdominus and lumbar multifidi. The transversus abdominus originates at the lower six ribs, thoracolumbar fascia, anterior three-fourths of the iliac crest, and the lateral one third of the inguinal ligament. It inserts into the linea alba, pubic crest, and pectin. (Department of Neurobiology and Developmental Sciences, 2009).

This muscle is activated upon exhalation. I used to laugh because some people go the gym and do lots of abdominal exercises focusing on the rectus abdominus, which if tight, as mentioned earlier, can compress the diaphragm. If you really are looking for a slim waistline and a strong core, the key is working on the transversus abdominus. Why? Because it has a direct connection to the diaphragm and the two work hand in hand.

Before I explain how to activate the transversus abdominus in your own body, I want to mention the importance of sound and sound therapy. Sound works directly through the connective tissue. Using your own voice to direct a muscle or body part to move activates the connective tissue directly. You have to move away from someone else telling you how to move and listen to your own voice because that is more powerful. Music can also play a role in muscle and body activation.

To find this valuable muscle, the transversus abdominus, I want you to find the anterior superior iliac spines which are bony projections of the iliac bone just beneath the abdomen on the front of the hip on both sides of your body. Take your hands and move them two inches down from there, and then face them inward as if your hands are in your pockets.

Now, you are going to use sound therapy to find this muscle. As your hands are on these areas, I want you to make the first sound, SHH. Did you feel the muscles pop into your hands? Try some other sounds like FFF, SSS, and even try coughing. Other clues that you can give someone to locate this area are "think, drawing in, bringing navel to spine, bring your pubic bone to your tailbone, pinch or pull your underwear in, or envision trying to zip up a tight pair of jeans" (Bond, M, 2007).

The lumbar multifidi, on the other hand, originates at the sacrum, transversus processes of C3-L5 and inserts on the spinous processes 2-4, vertebral levels superior to their origin. When these muscles contract on opposite sides of the spine, the spine will extend. When the muscles contract on the same side of the spine, it bends the spine in a side direction and rotates the spine in the opposite direction (Spencer, S, 2009).

This muscle is harder to locate then the transversus abdominus. Lie on your side with your leg bent and put your hand on your lower back. When you exhale, you might feel a slight plumping under your hand. It may feel like a sponge filled with water. If you can't feel it, use your SHH sound as someone pulls on your top leg slightly (Spencer, S, 2009).

Now that you are familiar with these muscles, remember to not get fixated on them. Our main focus should be on the breath and the movement of the diaphragm. Once the diaphragm is working correctly, then it will automatically connect to the transverse abdominis to the lumbar multifidi, creating a working team.

Muscles of the Trunk

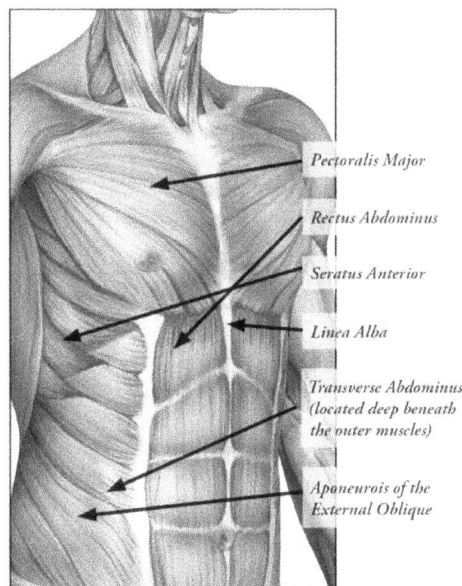

Pectoralis Major

Rectus Abdominus

Seratus Anterior

Linea Alba

Transverse Abdominus (located deep beneath the outer muscles)

Aponeurois of the External Oblique

Things to Think About

If a client has a pelvic floor dysfunction, the focus should be on the breath and diaphragm. If a client has lower back issues, you must evaluate the breath and the movement of the diaphragm first. Several studies have revealed that degeneration of the lumbar multifidi of the spine can be a result of poor posture and deactivation of the diaphragm. Clients with cervical spine or neck issues should also be evaluated for proper breathing, since the diaphragm is innervated by the phrenic nerve – C3, C4, C5. Focus on the breath.

When exercising, in addition to moving from this navel center point, I also want you always to keep your head in neck lock with all exercises. If someone has a visual impairment, poor balance, or is just unsure of how to perform a movement, they will most often look at the ground with their eyes. The ground provides stability and protection from falling. However, if someone's head drops or the chin moves to the chest, then most likely his or her shoulders will go forward. This is followed by dropping at the waist, thus compressing the diaphragm.

Neck lock actually opens the thyroid gland and opens the centers to the medulla oblongata, which is the respiratory center of the brain. Neck lock is simply bringing your chin towards your chest, keeping your head in neutral, and imagining that there's a rope from the top of the head to the bottom of your feet. You feel as though it's actually pulling, pulling, pulling you up so you can feel your cervical vertebrae lengthening.

An Exercise in Misalignment

I'm going to coach you through an exercise so you can perceive how it feels to be out of normal anatomical alignment and unable to perform functional activities. While performing this exercise, don't say anything. Just go within and listen. Focus on sensing what is happening within your body.

Sit in a chair and move your pelvis into a posterior pelvic tilt, like you are slouching. Okay, good. Now, continuing in the slouched position, lean your body all the way to the right side. Good. Stay in this position, and take your right shoulder and bring it slightly forward. Still staying in this position, now bend your head to the left side and rotate it to the right. Okay, excellent! Don't change this position. Just bring your right knee to your chest. Bring your leg down. And now bring your left knee to your chest. Bring this leg down. Lastly, within this same position, take your right arm and reach to your left side to touch your foot. You are done. Please return to a sitting position.

What did you feel like in these positions? Did they feel comfortable? Did you notice anything unusual going on in your body? What about your breath? Was it easy or difficult to breathe?

While performing this exercise, I hope you were able to witness how it feels to be in pain and unable to communicate your needs. Did you see the world differently because of the way you were holding your body? Could postural habits be related to some sensory imbalance, like vision or hearing or performance? Are tonal issues or the state of muscle tension really just related to postural problems?

My client population includes special needs clients from birth to 100 years of age. The majority of them are sitting in their wheelchairs for most of the day. I hate to say it, but most of their wheelchairs do not fit them correctly. Some of my clients are unable to talk or have visual issues. I will bet they are screaming inside from sitting long hours in their wheelchairs, but no one can hear or understand them. Similarly to Jello in a mold, their bodies conform to sitting in poor alignment. Once removed from their wheelchairs, their bodies stay in these conformed positions, whether placed on a mat or in a walking device. Their poorly fitted chairs and the lack of staff getting them out of their chairs throughout the day, has left them with muscle tightness, body neglect, constipation, respiratory issues, bowel and bladder dysfunction and either depression, anxiety, or anger. Why? Most likely because poor posturing within their chairs keeps their diaphragms compressed, limiting oxygen to the pelvis and back area and even to the brain. The result is limited functionality and inability for any type of independence.

The lesson is that we all have habitual patterns that we've had for a long time. Whether you're crooked like a person confined to a wheelchair or you are just habitually sitting slouched, it's still going to affect your breath and it's going to also affect your diaphragm.

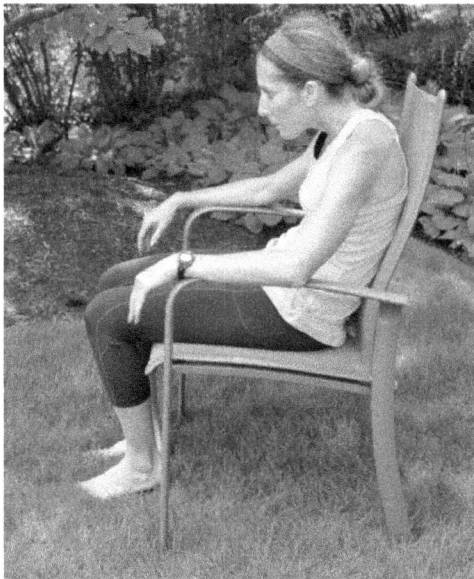

Improper Sitting

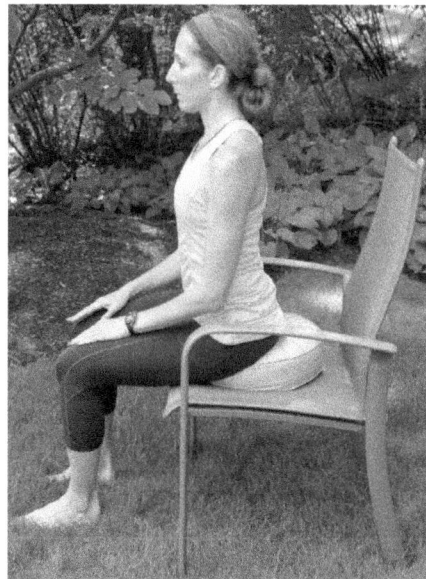

Proper Sitting using a Pillow

Chapter 4: Postural Knowledge - Connecting to Yourself

Yogi Bhajan often told people that age is not how old you are but rather how flexible you are. He said a 90 year old could be younger and healthier than a 20 year old solely due to flexibility.

Posture and the Stages of Life

Remember when you were a toddler playing outdoors. You had no worries or responsibilities. You were able to freely express through your body without any concerns or fears. You leaped, ran, jumped and enjoyed life, and your breathing was natural.

Now imagine yourself as a teenager in today's world. Self-esteem issues, peer pressure, guilt, rebellion, and lack of exercise from sitting and playing video games or working on the computer have left you with your head hanging down, your shoulders rounded and your chest depressing. Perhaps, your lung capacity is lessening. Look at one of today's fashions for teenage boys. They wear their pants so low on their hips that the crotch of the pant interferes with their walking and posture. Did you know that the origin of wearing your pants in that style came from the jails, where it meant that you were available?

Next imagine yourself in your 20's and 30's. Life is fun. You may have started a new job. You are exercising and enjoying life, but you're paying little attention to your body. As your duties and responsibilities in life become more demanding, you start to forget about the breath. You may notice your jaw hurts or you have neck and back pain, and you may have headaches.

You are in your 40's, 50's, 60's, and so on, and all the tolls of life have put a strain on your body. From sitting long hours at workstations or neglecting your diet and forgetting to exercise, you may now be experiencing sciatica, vision issues, bunions, or shoulder, neck, back and jaw issues. Your muscles have become tighter. The muscles that control the thorax which help with inhalation have also become tense, restricting exhalation. Your circulation slows down and your breathing changes creating all kinds of problems (Bond, M., 2007). And you're asking yourselves why your body seems to be falling apart.

A good example of this scenario is my father who just retired after fifty years in dentistry. Since he retired, he has had a variety of problems, from hips to shoulders to hand shakiness to degenerative changes within his spine and overall pain. Think about the physical demands of his profession. A dentist has to lean over his patients all day, using small tools to clean and check peoples' mouths. The contorted, flexed posturing and the delicate fine motor skills needed to successfully perform his job haven't helped his breathing or his overall health status.

Did you know that 85 percent of Americans will experience low back pain sometime in their lives and that 75 percent of Americans spend most of their waking lives sitting behind a steering wheel or in front of their computer screen? (Bond, Mary, 2007) In fact, the leading cause of low back pain is poor posture.

Important Postural Trends

Three things within our society today have significantly impacted our posture. These are our driving skills, our workstations, and how we eliminate – yes, going to the bathroom. Let's look at each impact more closely.

The number one impact is how we drive. Think about it. Driving is stressful. You need to keep your eyes on the road because you never know what another driver is thinking about or what they might do. Today, there is a lot of road rage, so you need to be a more defensive driver on the streets.

Additionally, the majority of us are in a hurry all the time. As a result, we slouch in the driver's seat. We grab the steering wheel with our thumbs and index fingers and instantly our shoulders go forward, our neck goes forward, and our diaphragm compresses. It's impossible to have really good diaphragmatic breathing when we are sitting like this. If you sat upright and held the steering wheel with your ring finger and index finger squeezed together, your posture would change because your scapular or your shoulder blades would move together, bringing your spine into extension. That is because of the connective tissue connection from these fingers to your triceps and to your rhomboids.

Now, let us look at our workstations. Society is focused on technology. Our ability to communicate is now almost totally dictated through our phones and our computer systems. Actually, the frequency of having a face-to-face conversation with someone is diminishing.

Unfortunately, as a result of our computer and phone usage, the body has taken a hit. Sitting in a forward flexed posture has weakened our diaphragms. Think about it. People complain of headaches, jaw issues, and even carpal tunnel syndrome. It is a no brainer to figure out why? Fix your work station. For example, find an appropriate chair or sit on a Swiss ball that will stabilize your pelvis and place it in a slight anterior pelvic tilt. This will create a straighter spine and keep your neck in neutral alignment. Raise the desk height or computer so that your arms are at about a ninety degree angle, making your scapula or shoulder blades pull together. Learn how to breathe, and both your work and your life will become more enjoyable.

The third thing that has gotten us in postural trouble is how we eliminate – how we go to the bathroom. In other countries, some people do what is called squatting because of the lack of toilet facilities. Squatting opens up the pelvic floor, which automatically creates good diaphragmatic breathing.

In our society, how do we sit on the toilet? Unfortunately, our toilets cause us to sit in a posterior pelvic tilt, closing the pelvic floor and perhaps, worsening our ability to eliminate. This can cause constipation issues. If we are unable to eliminate, then toxins can build up in our system leading to many other ailments.

A simple solution to this problem is to add a stool under the toilet. This will raise your legs and create a somewhat squatting position, opening the pelvic floor. Good deep breaths and working the diaphragm can also help.

Let me share an example from my own experience. My son who is now four refused to sit on the toilet to eliminate. He had constipation issues. I didn't see anything wrong with him squatting in his diaper at a young age. Babies instinctively know what is right but society just has to change things. I don't think society does it to just be different. It is more adults in society often invent something that's supposed to be an improvement, but which is actually not as healthy as doing "what comes naturally." When I realized that it was time for him to really use the toilet, I put a stool in front of him so he could still squat. He was happy and so was I.

Women who give birth in modern hospitals are usually told to lie on their backs and push. Guess what? Standing and squatting will help open the pelvic floor easily and the breath can flow better to make for an easier delivery.

Why are there a lot of geriatric patients in the hospitals for pneumonia and constipation? It's because, of course, how they sit. They sit in a forward flexed posture, compressing their diaphragms. It is impossible to get good diaphragmatic breathing when you are bent forward. A simple solution would be to add a pillow under the tailbone area, which will create an anterior pelvic tilt at their pelvis, opening up their pelvic floor and extending their spines.

Mary Bond in her book, *The New Rules of Posture*, in 2007 reported that in studies of present day societies in which people squat rather than sit in chairs, researchers have discovered lower rates of spinal disc degeneration than in societies in which people sit in chairs. In America no person older than the age of four squats. Instead, Americans spend most of their time sitting in chairs with poor posture.

Creating a Healthy Body from the Inside Out

Today, everyone wants "six pack abs" or an ideal figure or shape. Healthy posture and breath is the avenue to an ideal shape. Change your focus from how you look on the outside to what is occurring within. By looking at postural change within and becoming aware of the breath, you will develop within yourself a new awareness aligned with gravity which will help you feel balanced and taller.

Our society and we, ourselves are at fault for the way our posture and breath have changed over time. We all began in this world as nose breathers, but as we grow up, through habitual patterns, our diet, the environment, and the stresses and strains of life, we have changed our posture and breath. We were always taught that posture is just body alignment and unrelated to how we feel. But this new postural perspective applies to our own personal experience of living within our bodies and how we move in relationship to the world. It is the expression of our mind and body.

Posture and breath is also the association between our habits of movement, our pain, and our aging process. Posture and breath is a dynamic activity. It is created by our motions, how we hold ourselves and proceed through life, and how we were and are supported and regarded by other people from the time we were born and even in the womb. When we are in hurry all the time, our posture and breath follow this pattern. We breathe more quickly and less deeply.

Posture and breath are also shaped by our cultural and religious standards, by our geography, by the weather, by fashion, by stress, by media, by pollution, and most importantly, by our relationship with gravity. Additionally, we often hold ourselves and our bodies in response to some type of danger in our lives, to our emotions, or to memories. These threats are held as emotional patterns or protective reactions within our body and later show up as chronic tensions or habitual patterns (Bond, M, 2007).

As human beings, we are complex and deep creatures. Focusing and living on the surface level of life may hold us back from discovering the beauty and the gifts we hold inside. Our ignorance is like being in darkness, unable to clearly see the truth of our lives.

Physical Healing Involves More Than Just Body Positioning

With internal growth and awareness, we can grow toward the warmth of love and compassion and toward the light of truth. When we become well anchored with ourselves, we are able to handle the changing current of any situation. As we throw out our fears, emotions, judgments, and ego, we can become free.

So how do we do this? As a physical therapist, I always felt like a psychologist, but of course, I am not. The reason I say this is because my clients would always share their problems with me. Sometimes I would literally have to refer them to a psychologist because their emotional problems were held in their physical body. In fact, their physical pain was really psychological pain. The mind and the body connect!

It has only been during the last five years that our field has launched research on cognition and behavior. We are now addressing how our clients view their illness and their perceptions of their health by identifying negative thoughts. When we then challenge those negative thoughts, we can assist our clients to problem solve and devise coping plans using pleasant imagery. This new approach provides a more positive way to help people become more proactive about their pain and managing their pain, encouraging more patient-directed problem solving (Nielson, M, Keefe, F, Bernell, K, and Jull, G, 2014).

An interesting part of this new cognitive-behavioral approach is that simply teaching the client how to breathe correctly can open up the doorway to immediately discovering and resolving psychological issues. Emotional holding patterns can be released. A client may cry, get angry or scream. The therapist must hold the space for the client and play a supportive ego-free role in guiding the client to elevation.

How many of you can relate to feeling lost or unsettled within your body? Do you speak negatively about yourself or use vocabulary that doesn't support YOU! Do you consider your body as an **IT** instead of an **I**. Perhaps, your knee hurts and you point to the knee and say "that thing hurts me" or you may say "that darn arm." As you will discover, posture and breath requires you to be present within, honoring yourself – your entire being: mind, body, and soul.

Connecting with Your Body

In order to take the next step, you must begin connecting with your body. Imagine that two people are talking on the phone, and suddenly, the phone disconnects. The two people would not be able to finish their conversation which could have been important.

Now imagine that everything is connected within your body. You, for example, are trying to write your name on a piece of paper and suddenly the pen falls to the floor. How will you be able to write? How will you communicate with your body and create a reconnection to be able to speak to your body again?

For example, Mr. Jones, a client of mine, was in therapy because he suffered a stroke that resulted in his left side, especially his arm, being not functional. He was unable to feed himself or write his name and those tasks soon became his therapeutic goals. His brain, like the phone line, lost its connection to his hand. He needed to reconnect these two lines, both personally and with outside verbal cuing, so that functional movement could occur again. He needed to reconnect verbally, tactilely, visually, and through smell – aromatherapeutically. Verbally, he used positive self-talk with his hand to get it to move by "talking to it." Tactilely, he touched his hand, giving it love and support. Visually, he used his eyes to watch and direct his movements. To add an aromatherapy connection, I used an orange by simply cutting the orange in half and spraying the juices around the environment to help awaken and energize anyone within the area where it is sprayed. These components were essential to his recovery and reconnection.

Here is an example of how connecting with your body can create healing. Sarah, a client of mine who suffered a spinal injury could still feel her own body. She learned to control her spasms by internally moving herself in the direction that the spasm was already taking her. She turned the spasm into an intention. She would close her eyes and watch internally where the spasm was going, talking to her body and asking her body to please control the spasms by touching the spasming area with love and kindness. Guess what? Her spasms stopped, and she learned a way of reinterpreting what was happening inside of her by experiencing whatever was going on as if it was something she herself was doing.

Alternative Ways to Connect with Your Body

Take a brief moment and look at other ways you can connect with your sensory system.

Eyes: You can connect to your eyes by using color (more information on this later) or adaptive equipment, by closing your eyes and going within or by using a mirror to clearly see yourself. You can use the natural light of the sun for illumination and avoid fluorescent or luminescent lighting because these lights can emit a high frequency pulse, causing eye irritation which can bring on seizures with epileptic clients.

In 2014, the Consumer Energy Center published an article reporting that fluorescent lamps go on and off 60 times per second because of the cycle of electricity. Today, newer fluorescent lamps can cycle at 23,000 hertz, and no one can see the flicker. Thus, the brain can't be aware of something that changes so quickly. This in fact can be a good thing for some people. Fluorescent lighting can commonly cause drowsiness, migraines, and even some sympathetic responses associated with the perception of the flicker. (Seattle Community Network, 2007).

Touch: You can connect to your body by tapping (tapping the muscle that needs to become activated), using pressure points (reflexology or acupressure), by using equipment like hockey pucks and bean bags to bring awareness to an area or by using the heat of your hand. Working with the client's energy through Reiki also increases touch connection. Joint compressions at the joints cause stability, improved tone, and relaxation. Simply place your hands above and below a joint surface and slowly and gently bring your hands together, like a light squeeze. An example of this is weighted vests.

Joint Compressions

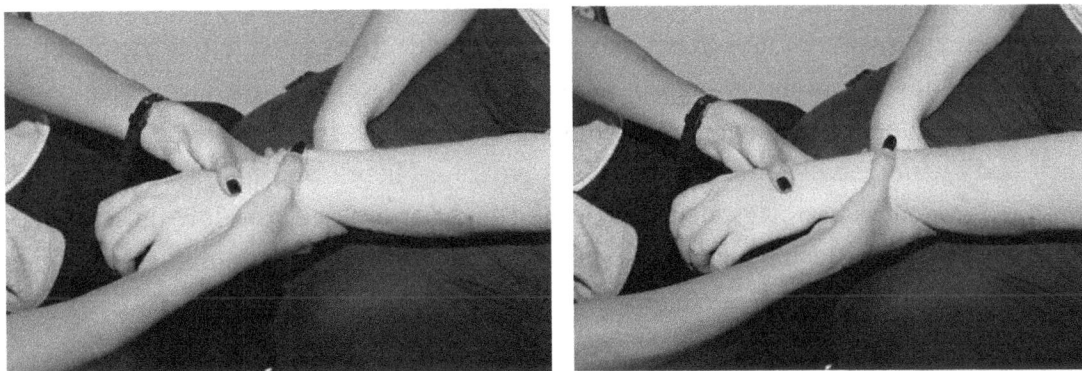

Auditory: To connect with your body through sound, use music, chanting, talking to yourself and your body or by getting verbal cues (sounds, voice, blowing) from someone else where the tone and vibration are altered as needed.

Proprioceptive: This is the body's ability to receive stimuli to detect the sensation of movement, position and balance. The system is made up of receptors in our muscles, joints, and connective tissue. It gives us information as to where our body is in space and how much pressure we use to grip things. It is referred to as "position sense." It provides information about range, force, and direction of movement. It contributes to muscle tone, posture, and equilibrium.

Examples of Exercises

For example, an exercise I use prior to getting my clients to walk is *Pawing*, a physical therapy technique, whereby I take their foot and move the foot through the motion of walking-heel-toe-push off. I repeat it reciprocally on each foot for about five to ten repetitions. Additionally, I incorporate having the client look at his or her foot and talk to it as they are going through the pawing motion.

I also perform another technique where I take their foot and slap it on the ground as though I was helping them with the marching motion. This provides immediate grounding and body awareness and initiates the nervous system to act. This is important to do prior to any walking training. If dizziness occurs with standing or any instability with walking, this will immediately prepare the body and ground it, decreasing the risks for falls and safety issues.

One last technique I created is called *Reawakening the Neglected Side.* The client is on his/her back or in the supine position. The therapist holds the client's leg and applies rhythmic oscillations or joint compression movements to the client's good side. The vibrations create a sense of movement on the affected side that can be felt by the client. The vibration overflows from the strong side of the body to the weaker side. It can then be done on the weaker side to strengthen the vibration, movement, and function. The client connects to their body with their eyes and voice. This is great for client's ability to feel movement or a sense of awareness to a neglected part of their body or an area with low muscle tone or muscle weakness. The technique can also just be done to the upper extremities.

Proprioceptive Techniques: 1. Grounding with heal/toe push off (Pawing) and 2. Reawakening the Neglected Side

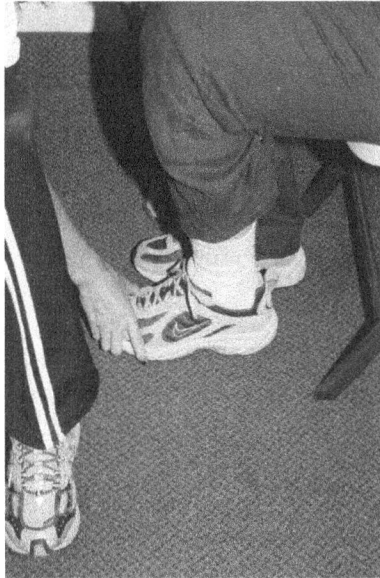

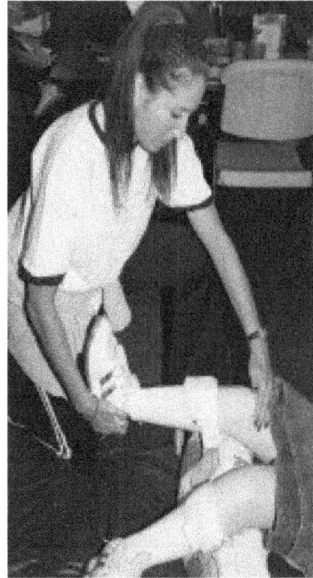

Vestibular: This is the sensory system known for helping with our balance and knowing our whereabouts in space to aid in coordinating our movements. It is located in the upper ear. It also signals changes in motion of the head through space and signals changes in position of the head with respect to gravity. It contributes to equilibrium, coordination of both sides of our body, and maintenance of muscle tone. Examples of ways to connect to the vestibular system include swinging, dancing, rolling, spinning, and even walking with bare feet.

Smell or Aromatherapy: Aromatherapy has been used for therapeutic purposes for nearly 6000 years. It works with the autonomic nervous system and utilizes pathways which promote endorphin release, neurotransmitter release, and regulation of blood pressure and breathing. It can be used for visual and auditory assistance.

The oils of aromatherapy are made from extractions from roots, leaves, seeds or blossoms of plants. I use natural smells in therapy directly from fruits, such as lemons and oranges. Certain oils can aggravate certain disorders. Avoid rosemary and cypress for high blood pressure. Some practitioners advise avoiding clove, cinnamon, sage, and hyssop during pregnancy.

Here are some of the most commonly used aromatherapy scents and their uses as excerpted from the following articles: "*Natural First Aid*," "*Illness Kit, Discovery Fit and Health*," and "*Aromatherapy*" (Keville, K, 2014; Kate, Wellness MAMA, 2013; and Seekers, J, 2011).

1. Lemon – Good for memory, work productivity; helps with circulation.
2. Rosemary/orang – Good for creativity.
3. Orange – Stimulating; good for awakening and creativity; can lower blood pressure.
4. Tea Tree Oil – Treats yeast infections, athlete's foot, insect bites, treats bacteria, fungi, and viruses.
5. Ginger – Stimulates appetite; anti-nausea.
6. Chamomile – Tension and insomnia.
7. Jasmine – Good for meditation.
8. Frankincense – Used to treat respiratory complaints; slows and regulates the breath.
9. Geranium – Harmonizes the emotions. Use it in a vaporizer to treat respiratory complaints or gargle with it to treat a sore throat. It is also good for skin care and for the female system, especially for new moms.
10. Cypress – Used to treat low blood pressure and poor circulation.
11. Eucalyptus – Used to treat flu, fever, and sore throat.
12. Peppermint – Helps digestion, arousal, vertigo, and nausea.
13. Lavender – Helps relaxation; good for pain and inflammation; attention deficit disorder; headaches; meditation; helps with sleep problems.
14. Grapefruit – Sexual attraction properties.
15. Rosemary/Frankincense – Stimulates appetite; good for poor circulation and fatigue.
16. Sandalwood – Relaxing and tonifying effect on the nervous system; promotes confidence.
17. Pine – Helps circulation. It can be made into a warming rub for muscular pain; helps with lethargy and listlessness
18. Chamomile – Speeds healing, calms inflammation and allergies, and treats burns, bruises, ear aches, toothaches. It has a calming effect; helps skin disorders; helps acid reflux.
19. Patchouli – Used for first aid treatment for minor burns because of its anti-inflammatory effect; calms nerves; is an aphrodisiac.
20. Hyssop oil – Good for arthritis, anxiety, bruises, respiratory infections, congestion, parasites and circulatory disorders. Increases low blood pressure and helps fight viral infections.

Good Habits for Increased Body Awareness

It is time to take the next step into really understanding what body awareness is and how to change our habits. The following exercise will help you link your sense of self with your sense of your body.

Exercise

Take a moment and attend to your body. Without altering your body, become aware of your body experience. What are the first sensations or tensions that you feel? Where are they? How are you breathing – quickly or slowly? What is your posture like?

Now ask yourself if you feel anything? You may say that you don't feel anything. Do you have a sense of self?

You may say, "Right now I notice that my breathing feels tight or shallow" or "Right now I notice . . ."

Begin to change your wording. Say instead, "I notice or I am connecting, or I am tensing my shoulders."

What happens during this shift? Did your breath become more diaphragmic? Did you feel grounded within your body as though a sense of peace and calmness surrounded you? Did your thinking become clearer? For those of you who immediately felt the connection to your body, try going deeper into the awareness by using the breath and see if you discover something more.

You may have witnessed this shift for yourself or you may be one that doesn't feel like attending to your body. Maybe you don't feel much of a connection with yourself and your existence or perhaps the way your body feels is trivial to you. If you had discomfort with this exercise, you may be experiencing a sense of meaninglessness or a lack of relationship to yourself. If this is the case, please continue reading this book to gain further assistance in building this important relationship between yourself and your body (Bond, M., 2007).

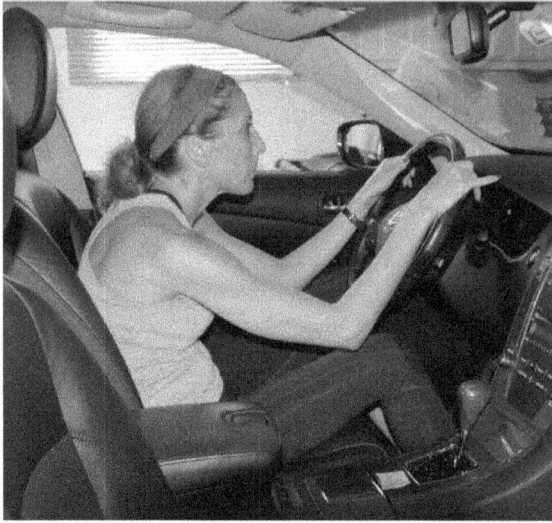

Improper Driving Posture

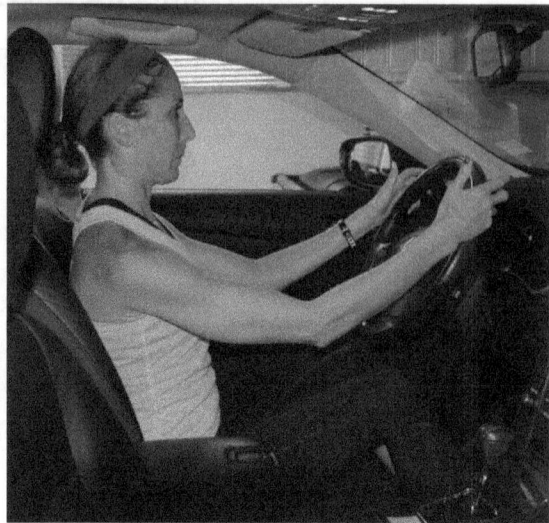

Proper Driving Posture

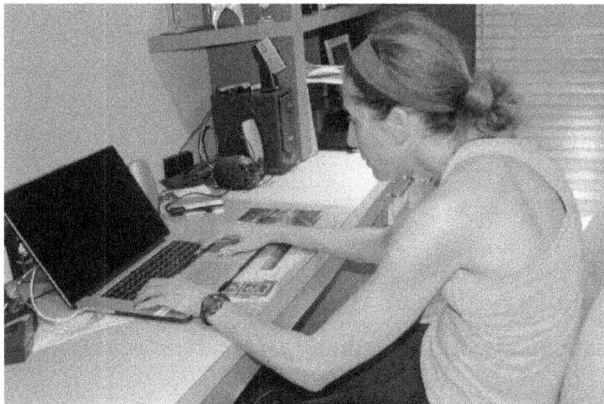

Improper Sitting Posture

Proper Sitting Posture

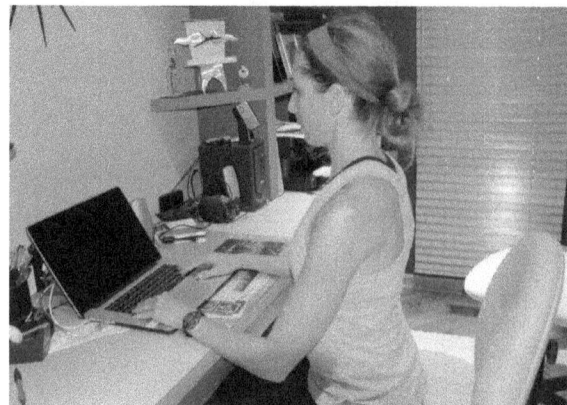

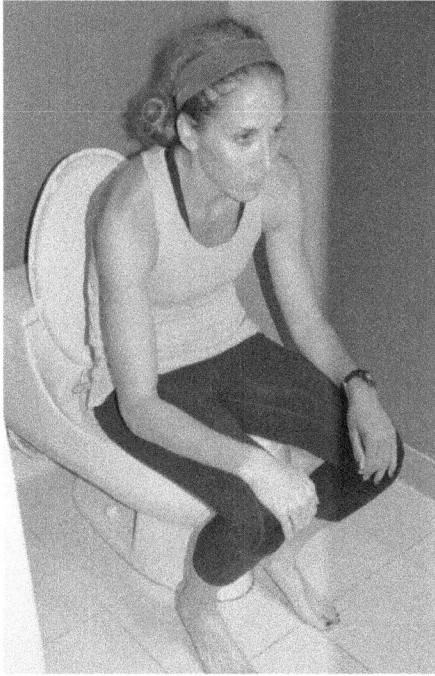

Improper Toilet Posture

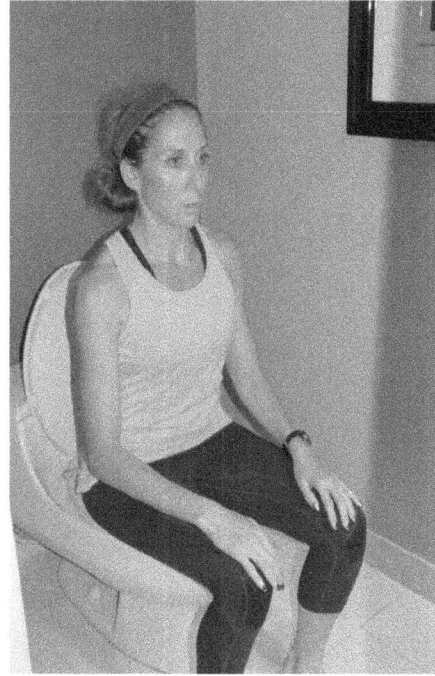

Proper Toilet Posture

Chapter 5:- Understanding Body Awareness: A Nervous System Perspective

"The kind of aware learning is complete when the new mode of action becomes automatic or even unconscious, as do all habits."
Moshe Feldenkrais

What do the words like weak or strong, hot or cold, tight or loose, soft or hard, tense or relaxed mean to you? Yes, they are opposites, but more importantly, these words are examples of terms used to help identify various bodily sensations. Whether a baby is crawling, an athlete is running, or a geriatric woman is walking with her walker, the question is, "Are these individual aware of their bodies?" Are you aware of your body?

What is Body Awareness?

Body awareness is defined as the "precise subjective consciousness of body sensations arising from stimuli that originate both outside and inside the body." (Rothschild, Babette, 2000) It involves receiving cues from the sensory system of the nervous system.

Stimuli for body awareness can come from either inside or outside of the body.

"Exteroceptors are nerves that receive and transmit information from the environment outside of the body (touch, taste, smell, sound and sight). Interoceptors are nerves that receive and transmit information inside of the body (connective tissue, muscles and viscera)." (Rothschild, Babette, 2000)

Body awareness is not an emotion, such as "I am afraid." Emotions are identified or interpreted from a blend of individual body sensations. For example, body awareness is not "I am frightened," but instead, "My breathing is shallow, my hands are cold and sweaty, and I feel like my heart is beating outside my stomach."

Understanding the Complexities of the Nervous System

Before I move on, I want everyone to understand how body awareness plays a role in the nervous system. In order to do that, it will be helpful to review the basic structure of that system. It will also be valuable to understand this system since it plays such a vital role in our behaviors and how we move and perceive the world.

The nervous system is divided into the Central Nervous System and the Peripheral Nervous System. The Central Nervous System is made up of the brain and spinal cord. The Peripheral Nervous System connects the central nervous system to the limbs and organs, serving as a communication link to many "systems" between the brain and the extremities.

As we have just learned, the Peripheral Nervous System is divided into the sensory and motor divisions. The sensory division is made up of the exteroceptive system and interoceptive system. The exteroceptive system consists of the five senses, or sensory nerves that respond to stimuli outside of the body. The interoceptive system is made up of sensory nerves responding to stimuli occurring inside the body.

Proproiception is one kind of interoception. Proprioception is made up of receptors in our muscles, joints, and connective tissue that give us information as to where our body is in space. Proprioception is commonly referred to as our position sense, and it contributes to muscle tone, posture, and equilibrium.

The vestibular system is another type of interoception. Our vestibular sense is our sense of balance and knowing our whereabouts in space. The vestibular sense contributes to our equilibrium and our spatial relation to the earth. Located in the inner ear, it signals any changes in the position of the head with respect to gravity. This is the part of the Sensory Nervous System, both interoceptive and exteroceptive, where we get the cues for body awareness.

The other part of the Peripheral Nervous System is the motor division. It is made up of the somatic nervous system and the autonomic nervous system. The somatic nervous system is under voluntary control. It is our conscious control. When we receive sensory input from the sensory division, our muscles and body can move, activating the somatic nervous system.

The autonomic nervous system is involuntary. It has no conscious control. It is regulated by the hypothalamus, a nervous system gland and an endocrine gland. (Rothschild, B., 2000).

The chart below may help remind you of the different levels of the nervous system and how they interrelate.

Levels of the Central Nervous System

1. *Central Nervous System*
   A. *Brain*
   B. *Spinal Cord*

2. *Peripheral Nervous system*
   A. *Sensory Division*
      (1) Exterocptive
      (2) Interoceptive
   B. *Motor Division*
      (1) Somatic Nervous System
      (2) Autonomic Nervous System
         (a) Sympathetic
         (b) Parasympathetic

The hypothalamus is a regulatory area for hormone concentration, thirst, hunger, body temperature, water balance, and blood pressure. It is associated with feelings of rage, aggression, hunger, and thirst. It also has connections with the pituitary gland -- the master gland that regulates secretions from the thyroid, adrenal, and reproductive organs. The pituitary gland produces hormones that influence blood pressure, contraction of the uterus, ovulation, bone maturation and growth, protein synthesis and the use of fat reserves. Moreover, the hypothalamus, which is the size of a walnut, is located below the thalamus, the relay station traveling to and from the spinal cord, brain stem, cerebrum, and cerebellum. The optic nerve even crosses at and intersects the connection between the pituitary gland and the hypothalamus. (Dale, C, 2009).

The autonomic nervous system is further divided into a sympathetic branch and a parasympathetic branch. These branches are involved in the fight or flight response. When an individual is stressed, the sympathetic branch will fire, increasing our breathing, heart rate and blood pressure and stimulating digestion. It will even dilate our pupils.

Our parasympathetic nervous system is responsible for bringing our bodies back into homeostasis or balance. When we are excited, we breathe through our mouths. Mouth breathing activates the sympathetic response, whereas nose breathing aids the parasympathetic response. It is important to keep this system – the autonomic nervous system – balanced for disease prevention. That is why the breath can help balance the body and the system and bring overall abundant health and wellness. Since stress is such a big factor in many people's lives, the autonomic nervous system is always being challenged to stay balanced.

Exercises to Enhance Body Awareness

Realize that you may or may not have a good sense of your body. You may be able or unable to communicate your body awareness to others. Some people are unable to feel their body sensations at all or they may not have the vocabulary to describe the sensations. Others may have little contact with their body, and when asked, may quickly switch the topic.

One way to understand body awareness is through your kinesthetic sense. This is where you place your body in a posture and ask yourself where a certain body part is positioned. For example, when you are standing, ask yourself, "Is my left foot weight bearing more than my right foot?"

Do you also consider your body to be something other than part of yourself? Being unable to connect to the "I" may be causing issues that prevent you from living a healthy and happy life. Because I am a physical therapist, those that seek help from me are usually the ones who actually want to get rid of some painful body experience. They want their pain to go away, yet they are often at odds with living and existing within their bodies. They may feel that looking at their body is wrong because of some past traumatic event like having been sexually violated. So, simply getting a client to attend to their body may open up an entirely new human experience. (Kepner, J, 1993). Conversely, the more we remove our identity from our own personal body experience, the more we become disconnected from society, suffering depression or other mental ailments.

Accessing the Body's Communication Systems

Walter Cannon did research and determined that that the body has its own wisdom to communicate. He found that since actual thoughts appear in the body, therefore physical activities can alter our thought patterns. He discovered that the simple act of breathing can change the type and quantity of peptides produced by the brain stem. Since many of the peptides in existence are known to originate in the respiratory system, then the simple activity of deep breathing can affect and calm the mind or help with anger and fear. (Khalsa, D.S., 2001).

Your voice commands your mind, body, and spirit. Energy plus vibration equal matter, and thoughts plus your voice equal reality. Phrases like "I can't" or "I won't" or any negative self-talk must leave your vocabulary and be replaced with statements like "I can, I believe, I can do it, I can do anything." These words directly connect you to the 'I" within you (Worldly Minds, 2013).

I recommend reading Louise Hay's book, *Heal your Body*. It is a wonderful book where Louise tells us to stop blaming others for what is wrong in our bodies and life. She explains how the power of our words and thoughts can create our experiences. She helps create healing affirmations based on the emotional cause behind the disease. For example, she says that if you suffer from anxiety, you may not be trusting the flow and the process of life. She gives an affirmation to say: "I love and approve of myself and trust the process of life" (Hay, L, 1982).

Using Louise Hay's suggestions, the first thing I ask my clients suffering from back issues are questions about money and support. These questions provide me with a starting point to discover an emotional cause that may be creating a physical manifestation within the body.

Recently, a friend of mine who is a firefighter came to see me for help because he had thrown out his back. As a result, he could hardly walk. Apparently, he had worked with another physical therapist who focused on Ultrasound and stretching treatments, but he claimed that they weren't able to alleviate his pain. My friend is a muscular man who presented himself with forward flexed posturing because of the extreme pain he was experiencing.

During the start of our treatment, I presented him with two questions: was he feeling supported and was he feeling financially supported. To my surprise, he spoke immediately about the fear of not making the firefighter captain position – an intense process to go through, the fear of not having enough money for retirement, and his marital problems at home. Our therapy session consisted of breath work, postural correction, and positive self-talk and positive declarations throughout the session, affirming that it is safe to live and to love life. After this one session, my friend walked out a new man, with a new posture and a new outlook on life.

Besides Louise Hay, there are other ways to connect with the "I" in your body. Kelly Ballard in September 2012 wrote an amazing article titled "Laugh your way to Better Health." She reports that studies have shown that laughter and telling a good joke have many medical and psychological benefits. She describes ten of these healing modalities for better health. They include assisting in weight management, slowing aging, helping with stress relief, increasing immunity, enhancing circulation, lessening risk of cancer; decreasing pain, managing diabetes, improving breathing, and exercise.

Another way to reconnect to your self is by making a dream board or vision board which consists of cutting out pictures or words that represent what you want to become or do in your life. You use them to make a collage on a piece of paper. Hang this paper somewhere

where you see it every day. This way you can make the dreams become reality and appreciate the part of you that is ready to grow and change.

Each moment of your life should become a dialogue of response and change. As Bonnie Bainbridge Cohen wrote, "Imbalances aren't weaknesses but strengths. If there is a point of weakness, don't become trapped on the place of stress or the problem. For example, if you have a shoulder problem, instead of seeing the weakness at the shoulder, see it as a result of forces that are converging on the shoulder from other places in the body. Thus, the shoulder may become a gift for you or a point of entry for you to discover the true cause of the problem."

She also says to align your inner cellular movement with the external expression of movement through space. Aligning within your body is not the goal. It is the dialogue between your awareness and action. This alignment will create a state of knowing. She continues to say that the ways to working toward alignment can be through movement, art, music, meditation, and through verbal dialogue (Bainbridge, C, 2012).

Sharing a Personal Experience

As another example of the power of thoughts and words, in my yoga practice we use mantras – a sacred utterance or a word or group of words with meaning. One word used is Sat Nam which means true identity. This word is chanted or said silently or even whispered when performing a yogic posture. You can combine it with breath by inhaling on the word "Sat" and exhaling on the word "Nam." Combining breathing with yoga postures reminds us of the importance of using breath with movement.

I want to just tell you a story of how this relates to my life. You already know I am a physical therapist, but I was also a professional in-line speed skater. I won't bore you with all the details, but in 2000 I was taken out in a race by a pack of girls and I ended up breaking my left wrist.

This happened in Minnesota. I had to have surgery in a hospital with doctors I did not know and with no family nearby. When I returned to Arizona, I couldn't find a doctor who would take over my case. Lots of doctors did not want the liability. I finally found a doctor who treated with professional athletes who would work with me. He looked at my report and told me that the doctor who had performed my surgery in Minnesota was, ironically, a friend of his from medical school.

The point I want to share with you is that my left hand got worse. It started turning blue and I was diagnosed with Reflex Sympathetic Dystrophy, a syndrome of unknown cause with symptoms of swelling, pain, and vascular dysfunction. The doctor literally scolded me and said in so many words, "You are a physical therapist. You need to work on your wrist." After pain clinic and medications, I came to my own resolution: "Practice what you preach." I had disconnected myself from my body because of this painful, traumatic experience. I was afraid I wouldn't be able to use my hand for physical therapy or for sports again

So I made a conscious effort to reunite with my body. I spent days looking at my hand, and massaging it. I kept talking with my hand, saying all positive affirmations and even letting go of all my fear. With deep conscious breathing, I eliminated my problem and dissolved all the negative attachments I had to this experience. Once this all took place, my hand began to heal.

It is time to let go of your habits. Yogi Bhajan said, "Habit is a must of your personality and mind. For that period when you are acting under a demoting habit, you are totally in the negative personality. It is also a fact that if you get into any one negative habit, you will automatically attract its four sister habits, for they love to stay together. These five demoting habits of behavior and attitude are greed, anger, lust, attachment, and negative ego. When one sister enters the house, she calls the others to join. Each habit is supported on two tripods- Physical, Mental, and Spiritual and Past, Present, and Future" (Bhajan, Y, 2000). In our yogic practice, Yogi Bhajan used to say it takes 40 days to change a habit, 90 days to confirm a habit, 120 days to develop the new habit in you, and by 1000 days, you have mastered your new habit (Bhajan, Y, 2007).

Are you ready to transform your life?

Chapter 6: Missing Links in Standard Assessments and Evaluation Tools

"Truthfully, the most important thing in life is knowing what the most important things in life are, and prioritizing them accordingly."
Melchor Lim

What components may physical therapists or health care professionals be missing as part of their standard observations, assessments, and evaluations? Because I am physical therapist, I evaluate range of motion, strength, transfers, balance, coordination, bed mobility, and ambulation. However, there are three missing links that should be performed by any health care professional when interacting with their clients. These missing links are posture, vision, and the breath.

Posturally, you can obtain a lot of information by how a client stands, sits, and moves around his or her environment. Sometimes you can observe what a client is not saying or use your sensations relating to them just by observing how they physically present themselves to you.

Eighty present of our sensory system is connected to our vision system. Recall that all the input we need to put our bodies into motion originates from our sensory system. Therefore, vision – a crucial part of our sensory system for most people – must be functioning efficiently. The vision system also tells us about the tonality of the entire body.

For example, if a client who had a stroke has difficulty moving the left side of his body, before any type of movement should occur, a visual assessment should be executed, preferably by an eye doctor. If there is a visual problem, then most likely the client will have difficulty moving. If I was this client's therapist I would anticipate that the client will present with upper and lower extremity neglect to the side of the visual deficit. He will be afraid to move because of the loss of visual perception and have difficulty with his/her balance and coordination. My job becomes easier if the visual deficit can be corrected prior to the initial evaluation.

The Importance of Vision for Movement

I was taught this understanding about ten years ago when I visited a developmental optometrist. Most of my clients have special needs. Researchers are finding that visual deficits can occur with clients diagnosed with Cerebral Palsy, Down's Syndrome, and Autism. Prior to engaging in conversation, the optometrist insisted that in order to have a full understanding of our meeting, she could perform a demonstration on me.

She sat me in a chair and put prism glasses on me – glasses to change my visual perceptions. She informed me that I was to pretend that I was a client who just had a stroke on my right side, and that I was to stand up and start walking. I attempted unsuccessfully three times to even stand up. I sat back down and told her I was unable to do this activity. I literally could not see anything out of my right eye. It felt as though I was blind in my right eye and had only one side to operate from – the left side. The thought of standing was scary because I had lost my connection to my body. Afraid and stunned, I replied I understood now the importance of vision. She laughed and asked me if I had gained more compassion for my clients in this three minute exercise.

Of course, I was fascinated by this discovery of the importance of the visual system. I asked her what she could do to help me if I had experienced a vision loss in the right eye. Treatment can simply be building up the eye muscles affected. Moreover, placing clients in prism glasses can help to correct visual deficits so they can see and connect with their bodies.

I was blessed, of course, by our meeting and the experience, and thankful that it had changed me as a person and as a therapist. Now when I see clients, I observe their eyes during our initial meeting. I also perform visual tracking exercises, observe their eyes reading, and observe their eyes when moving. I will go more into depth on the visual system shortly.

Evaluating Breath

The last component that I evaluate is the breath. If you have read the first two chapters of this book, then you already know that evaluating the breath is a mandatory task because the breath connects with everything within our body. Without them being aware of me watching, I observe how the client is breathing when they are sitting and standing and even while walking. After I have observed their normal breathing, then I ask the client to breathe for me in sitting and in standing positions and evaluate if they are a paradoxical breather – where the chest wall goes in on inhalation and out on expiration, the opposite of normal breathing – or just not really using their full lung capability. Lastly, I watch them walk and breathe. During this process, I observe where the stress is in their body and if their breath is fast, slow, and controlled.

Did you know that doctors can now administer a test called the ANSAR (Ansar Group, Inc., 2014), designed to determine the ability of both branches of the autonomic nervous system to respond to and relax from a challenge. This test can detect early dysfunction, correct the imbalance, and stop the progression of inflammatory disease, cardiovascular damage, emotional dysfunction, and nervous system disorders. Guess what tool is used as part of the test? The breath. Activities include deep breathing, holding the breath and bearing down lightly, and standing while breathing all while hooked up with ECG electrodes, a blood pressure monitoring system, a computer, and a technician to guide the client through each step of the test.

Postural Evaluation and Alignment

In the physical therapy profession, we have traditionally been focused more on posture as outer alignment rather than inner alignment. Outer alignment can be observed and corrected both verbally and hands-on or with the assistance of someone else's eyes, in this case the physical therapist. A typical postural exam is described by looking at the gravity line through an individual's body. This gravity line is considered "an ever changing reference line that responds to the constantly altering position during upright posture. The closer a person's postural alignment lies to the center of all axes, the less gravitational stress is placed on the soft tissue components of the support system. When a force couple, a pair of muscle forces that work together on a joint to yield rotation and can apply pulls in opposite directions, is out of balance, the segment moves off its axis of rotation and there is poor joint motion" (Epler, M, 1990 and Palmer, L, 1990).

As you have read from previous chapters, poor posture can be caused by numerous things, especially poor habits, aging, and our movement patterns. Unfortunately, people with structural scoliosis, irreversible lateral curvature of the spine with fixed rotation of the vertebrae, aren't fortunate enough to be able to ever resume normal spinal alignment unless corrected through surgery or bracing.

With structural scoliosis, the spinous processes of the vertebrae – the pointy things sticking out of your back along the entire length of your spine – rotate away toward the concave side of your body, whereby the rib cage can merge closer to your hip bone. This is also known as the shortened side. The vertebral bodies, on the other hand, rotate toward the convex side of the curve. A rib hump will occur on the convex side of the curve caused by the rotation of the vertebrae and the rib cage. So, compression of the ribs will be seen on the concave side of a structural scoliosis individual and separation of the ribs will be observed on the convex side, along with prominence of the ribs and scapula posteriorly.

Keep in mind, that there is another form of scoliosis, called nonstructural scoliosis, which can be corrected. It usually results from tight muscles causing one side of the body's muscular skeletal system to become very tight while the other side remains loose, bringing the body out of alignment and balance. Positioning is essential for both types. However, with structural scoliosis, it is important to keep the concavity or shortened side open so the diaphragm will not compress. A recommended position in this case is a sideline position – lying opposite of the shortened side.

Structural Scoliosis: The rib cage hitting the left hip bone.
Best position to open this side is placing the client on right sideline.

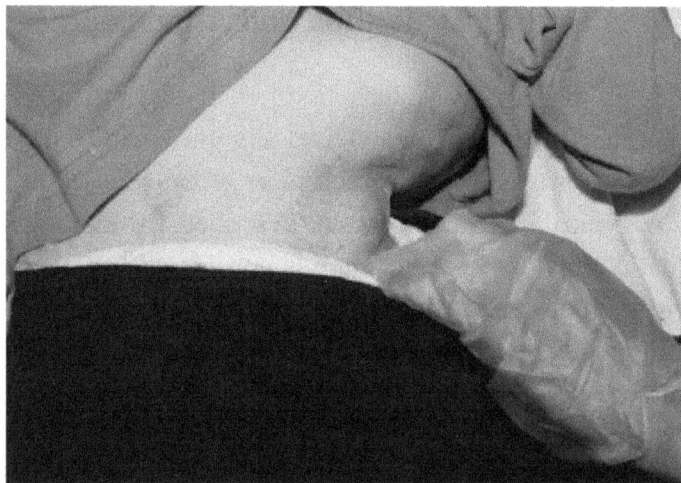

In most cases, and especially with my clients who have special needs, posture and positioning are of the utmost priority. I always make sure that a client's head, shoulders, hips, knees and feet are in correct alignment. Those of my clients who sit in wheelchairs for the majority of the day need to be taken out of their chairs and aligned. This is a mandatory activity because if not positioned correctly, over time the client may develop respiratory, bowel and bladder issues, not to mention many other health problems. Achieving this alignment can require pillows, bolsters, or other equipment.

Postural alignment involves imagining that a straight line is drawn from the top of a client's head to the bottom of his/her feet, dividing the body into two equal halves. In this process, you can notice if one shoulder is higher or more rotated than the other; if the head is rotated or tilted; if there is equal arm space between each arm; if there is equal weight bearing through the feet; if both of the arches are the same; if the hips are aligned or rotated; and so on throughout the observation. I call this my standing postural assessment test, where the client stands against a clean, non-distracting wall, and the therapist can visually pick up on any of these bodily changes.

Standing Postural Test

Do you see any differences between the right and left side of her body?

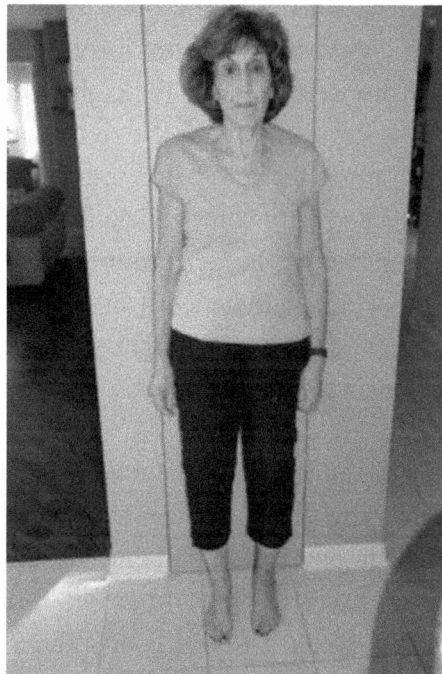

A strong indication of musculoskeletal changes within the body can be observed by looking at the fascial pull on both sides of the face, especially near the eyes, and even along the umbilicus or belly button area. Now before you run to the mirror and check out your body and get crazy, let me finish. It really is an interesting observational tool and can give you information on what is happening within your body.

If a client presents with a back issue, you might witness the connective tissue pulling around the eye region. For example, a golfer came to see me with a back issue. Before he was able to tell me what was wrong, it was written all over the fascial pathways of his eyes and around his umbilicus area. He presented with back problems on his right side, which gave me some indication that he probably swung his golf clubs using more of the right side of his body. What would you guess the fascial pathways around his eye and umbilicus area looked like? Of course, the right side of his face was tighter, giving an appearance of his eyes not being aligned. Around his belly button area, his umbilicus on the right was pulling more toward his right psoas muscle – a muscle that originates on the transverse processes of T12-L5 and inserts into the lessor trochanter of the hip – also giving an unequal appearance. His left umbilicus area showed a looser skin tone. With the umbilicus pulling to the right, the right side of his diaphragm muscle was also tighter.

Here is another example. I was teaching one of my courses on posture and scoliosis, and a therapist presented her personal case to the class. She told the class that she had been a speed skater for twenty years and, as a result, had major back issues. Looking at her fascial pathways, her face and her whole body were pulling to the right. I could almost feel her pain. When the class acquired more information about her speed skating career, she said that she skated in circles toward the right, which meant this continuous habitual motion required her body to lean toward the right with her right arm stabilized behind her back, while her left arm was used for momentum. Of course when skating the rink's straightaways her body got some relief. It was no wonder why this woman was having the problems she was having. In fact, from this prolonged activity, her head position was side bent to the right, which automatically created stress along her entire fascial pathway on her right side. I hypothesized that her right shoulder, right hip, right knee and right foot would also be affected as indeed they were discovered to be upon assessment.

Speaking of sports, athletes like me who have been running for many years will frequently experience tight hamstrings. If the hamstrings are tight, then the pelvis ends up in a posterior pelvic tilt, and the diaphragm will get compressed or the body will be limited in oxygen and endurance. Running is an art form and postural techniques are an essential component to this sport. To be a good runner requires body awareness and proper body alignment.

Umbilicus Photo: Fascia pulling to left side

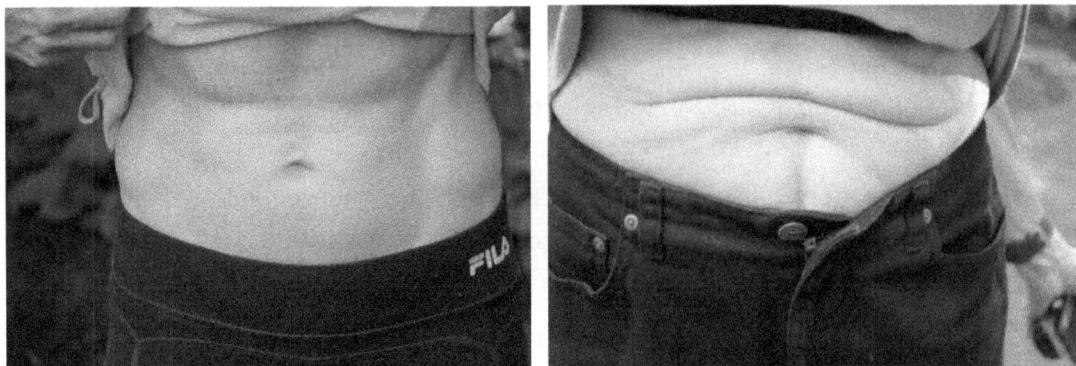

Fascia around the yes- Fascia pulling to left side

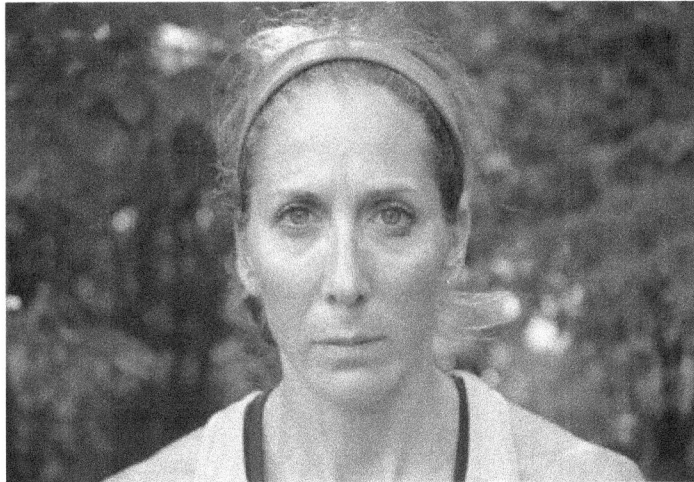

Keep in mind that postural changes almost always occur in special client populations, like the geriatric population and even with pregnant woman. As we age, our spine goes through degenerative changes, and medical issues may occur. Unfortunately, our posture may change. The head may move forward, the shoulders may round, and the pelvis may move more into a posterior pelvic tilt. Encouraging seniors to sit on chairs with cushions under their buttocks for support will help open the pelvic floor and bring the spine in a more neutral position. Neck lock exercises will also be beneficial to help bring the head and neck in better alignment.

With pregnant women, the weight of the baby may cause the lower back to sway as the center of gravity moves forward. The abdominal muscles may become stretched and contract less as the baby grows. Hormonal levels increase and therefore, joints and ligaments may loosen. Working on pelvic tilts, Kegel exercises, neck lock, and squatting can help improve these postural changes.

There are many muscles and nerves involved in achieving good postural alignment and respiration. If one muscle is tight in your body, imagine how it can create tension or stress somewhere else within the body. The whole body is connected through fascial pathways.

There are also many factors to consider that may cause postural changes besides age, our habits, and our movement patterns. One factor to consider is surgeries: past surgeries and recent surgeries. Any surgery may cause some type of compensation pattern somewhere else within the body, throwing off postural alignment. How a client views the illness may change his or her alignment. The type of work a client does may also be an issue. Is the client moving a lot throughout the day, doing repetitive work activities or sitting at a desk? Athletes, depending on the type of sport in which they are engaged, acquire specific and repetitive movement patterns which will create postural habits. For example, swimmers may have tight shoulders from overuse, creating more rounded, forward shoulders and tight neck musculature.

Smokers may also have issues because they are exhaling smoke out of their mouth and decreasing oxygenation to their lungs. As a result of this habit, smokers develop forward head and shoulder posturing and diaphragmatic compression. Take a moment and pretend you are blowing out candles on your birthday cake. What is your posture doing when you are performing this activity?

What about telephone users? Think about it? When we are talking on the phone, if not using a hands-free device, our head is often tilted and forward. Eventually, the constant tilting of the head will throw off alignment on the side you're talking on. The shoulder will soon drop, along with the hip, and your feet will change how they strike the ground.

Trauma or whiplash and even psychological issues, like depression, can alter how we stand and move. Wearing dentures, orthotics, heel lifts, having a congenital short or long leg, and postural abnormalities like scoliosis, orthopedic and neurological deficits should also be evaluated when looking at posture. Even those who have gone through stressful life changes, like divorce or drug and alcohol problems, may hold their bodies differently. Lastly, repetitive gum chewing can create tension within the jaw which creates problems within the entire body.

The Role of the Jaw in Posture

Let's talk about the jaw. It is one of the most complex joints in the body. One of the core fascial connections is the jaw's connection to the diaphragm, psoas muscles, pelvic floor, medial part of knee, and plantar part of the foot. Did you know that ninety percent of musculoskeletal issues have an element of TMJ involvement to them (Exeter Natural Health and Personal Development Blog, 2010)? The TMJ or temporal mandibular joint is the joint of the jaw that connects the jawbone to the skull. It is like a sliding hinge. Jaw issues may even represent emotional holding patterns. Headaches, neck and shoulder pain, swelling on the side of the face, dizziness, vision problems, and ringing in the ears are just some signs and symptoms of this disorder (TMJ and MFR).

It is important to restore balance throughout the entire body because the jaw has fascial connections to the majority of muscles within the body, especially to the psoas, glute, quadratus lumborum, and piriformis. These muscles must be treated. Other muscles to be worked are the upper trapezius, the neck muscles, and of course, all the jaw muscles.

Excessive gum chewing and mouth breathing, as mentioned above and as cited by Travell and Simon, can cause trigger points in the temporalis, one of the muscles of mastication or chewing. Referred pain from the trapezius muscle may also result in trigger points to the jaw area (Gallagher, M, 1990). In fact, forward head position can influence mandibular positioning and masticatory dysfunction (chewing difficulties). Imbalance in the pelvis, a fallen arch, a tight psoas muscle, an externally rotated femur, a medially and anterior rotated shoulder, atlanto-occipital compression, and other imbalances can make lines of pull throughout the fascial network that will directly affect the jaw.(TMJ and MFR).

The muscles of mastication are a group of muscles associated with movements of the jaw. There are four muscles of mastication: the masseter, the temporalis, the medial pterygoid, and the lateral pterygoid. The masseter is the most powerful muscle of mastication. It helps to elevate the mandible or jaw and helps to close the mouth. The temporalis elevates the mandible, closes the mouth, and can pull the jaw posteriorly. The medial pterygoid muscle elevates the mandible and closes the mouth. Lastly, the lateral pterygoid muscle protracts the mandible, pushing the jaw forward. Unilateral action creates the side to side movement of the jaw (Jones, 2014).

In order to see the pterygoids, you must cut the skull in half. Do you remember the sphenoid bone? That is the bone that looks like a bird that is kind of flying inside the skull. The pterygoids, the muscles of the jaw that provide elevation and lateral deviation, attach to the sphenoidal plate. The sphenoid articulates with 14 major skull bones and its function is to move rhythmically, like the wings of a bird, beating the craniosacral fluid around the skull. Based on its location, this bone is important for hormone production and regulation, the flow of nutrients both to and from the brain, and the whole nervous system. Because of its attachment to the Occiput bone or base of the skull bone, the rhythmic movement of these two bones together supports movement of these fluids, nutrients, and information within the central nervous system (Schell, S, 2001). These two bones can become dysfunctional from a variety of reasons, one being from jaw imbalances or TMJ.

If there is dysfunction, any movement can create an abnormal pull through the sphenoid bone affecting cranial structures which will affect the fluid movement of the vital craniosacral system (TMJ and MFR). This is an interesting concept because if someone has a jaw issue, it will not only affect all the muscles just mentioned, but all the bones and their attachments. Additionally, it will affect the craniosacral fluid that affects our nervous system. Any pull or tension in the jaw area is going to shift some part of our body in a certain way.

Lastly, the most common underlying cause of TMJ dysfunction and pain stems from an emotional component. There is an actual physical neurological link between the sensory (as well as the motor) nerves within the TMJ itself, which also links the brain and spinal cord via a branch of the Trigeminal nerve. These sensory mechanoreceptors, which are type 3 and type 4, will be discussed later in detail. Any type of emotional stress can cause the muscles of the TMJ to clench or tighten up, increasing the firing of the sympathetic nervous system. Learning yoga or relaxation and meditation techniques can be quite helpful for this problem (Exeter Natural Health and personal Development Blog, 2010).

It is time to begin your own personal exploration. In the next chapter, you will have the opportunity to experience different aspects of body movements. Try each movement so that you can really connect with your body. Remember, that through the experience, you will gain knowledge.

Chapter 7: Movement Exploration

"If your inner life is not producing what you would like on the outside, don't be discouraged . . . just be willing to change."
Joyce Meyer

Your Personal Exploration of Movement

I'm about to take you through your own movement exploration. We will be looking at many parts of the body, and even some habitual movement patterns we do every day of our lives. It might be beneficial to read a section and then try to do the activity. Be prepared that it could take one, two, or even three tries on your own to master each section. You may have to just keep practicing. It is through experience that you will gain the most knowledge. Let go of all your insecurities and go within.

The idea of this section is to focus on the breath and how it utilizes the core connection. If you are trying and attempting these exercises to the best of your ability, you will find a new sense of freedom within your body. It may take one or two times of practice to truly and honestly feel these new body experiences. Have fun!

Getting to Know Your Jaw

Let's begin by clenching your teeth and really sensing your jaw muscles contracting. Now, as you clench your teeth, try to focus on your nasal breathing and notice if the breath is staying in your chest and neck area or if it working the navel area as well as the chest and neck area.

Now relax your jaw and teeth. Feel like you are almost dropping the jaw – as if all the muscles of the jaw are being stretched or pulled downward. Breathe in and out of your nose, and notice if there is a difference? Is it easier this way to breathe and really fill your navel area?

Since the jaw is part of so many fascial pathways, keeping the jaw relaxed or dropping the jaw should be integrated into how you move and behave on a daily basis. Think of it like this: any pull or tension on the jaw is going to shift some other part of your body in some way. Most likely, it won't be for the best.

This idea of dropping the jaw was imprinted in my mind when I was delivering my son. One of the biggest things that a mother in labor should be told is to drop the jaw. Labor is not a pretty sight for those viewing it. It is painful for mothers like me who decide to give birth without medication. The moment pain hits the body, the body naturally becomes tense, especially the jaw.

Remember that the jaw has a connection to the pelvic floor. The pelvic floor needs to open and dilate for the baby to come out. By clenching the jaw, the pelvic floor doesn't open easily and labor and pain can be prolonged. Just a little reminder for mom's giving birth, save yourself lot of pain and time and relax your jaw. Have your partner or friend who is at your birth use this reminder to coach you through this process. Also, remember to stand and squat!

Clenching your jaw

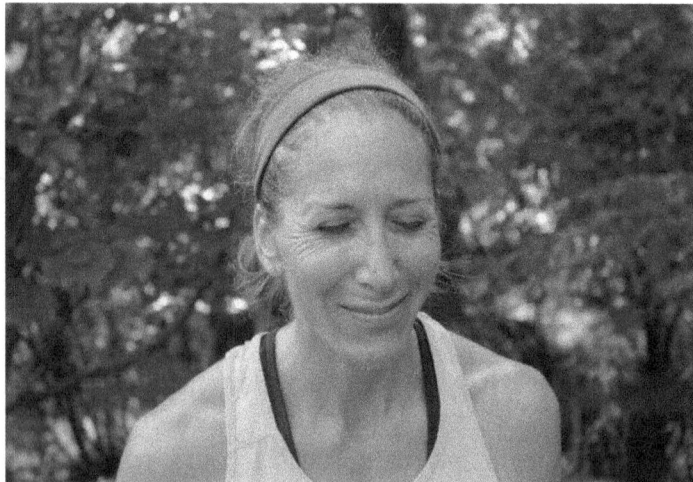

Getting to Know Your Shoulders

Bend your elbows to about 90 degrees. Hold your arms in this position and bring your shoulders up to your ears. Stay in this position. It is very uncomfortable, but just continue holding it. While you are in this position try to nasal breathe, breathing in and out of your nose with pursed lips. Focus on conscious breathing. Are you able to really fill up the navel area or is your breath restricted to the chest area.

A lot of runners keep their arms held tight like this during training and racing. Do you think these runners are the best endurance athletes with this positioning? Running, like any sport, takes training and learning proper body techniques. Runners who hold their arms rigid like this end up extending their neck and body. They are constantly resisting gravity, and therefore, their breath is centered in the chest area. Their stride length also becomes diminished.

There's a simple solution. Drop the arms, relax the shoulders, and imagine that you are gently holding a penny between your thumb and index finger. Your breath will naturally move to the navel area and your stride length and body positioning are now working with gravity and not against it. This is a winning resolution.

I see this stressful holding pattern quite frequently with my client population. This is called high tone. Tone is a state of normal muscle tension. Clients with high tone have increased stress or tension to any resistance within their environment. So, for example, a loud noise or trying to extend a client's arm would create even more resistance or tightness, making the individual prone to changes in the body in other areas. Increased shoulder tension can create side bending in the neck, which could then create a dropped hip, an internally rotated knee, and even a foot that is everted or turned outward. Changes all the way down in the fascial plane can take place. Most importantly, the breath becomes restricted.

Imagine yourself struggling with tension and stress within your body all day long, all week long, and even every day of your life. Anything within the environment can make it worse. Learning and performing some nervous system techniques on individuals with high tonal issues can help in the client's relaxation process and aid in moving the client's breath to the navel and pelvic floor area. As mentioned earlier, constipation and respiratory issues are big problems with hypertonic clients. Range of motion is not the key.

Neurotherapeutic techniques such as pressure on the tendon or pressure on the muscle belly itself will work the Golgi tendon organ which is a mechanoreceptor responsible for decreasing tone. These organs function as a protective mechanism in situations in which a muscle is elongated beyond its physiologic limits. For example, a muscle tear may be prevented by the relaxation of the muscle provided by the reflex action of the Golgi tendon organ.

Any muscle that is tight – in this case, the bicep muscle – can be released. Simply hold the bicep muscle of the client or the tendon of the muscle belly where these goji tendon organs are located. Use light gentle pressure-the amount of pressure used to grip a pencil. Keep your hands on this muscle or tendon. The client's eyes may look up as if trying to discover the source of this stimulus. The stimulus will go to the client's brain and create a relaxation response of the muscle, given the Golgi tendon organ is held. When the client eventually lets go, the therapist can lower the client's arm, pain free. The key is to keep pressure on this spot. This can also be done at the hamstring area to release tight hamstrings, along the adductors to help open up the legs, and most other areas of the body.

Once the release takes place, the client will become so relaxed that they might fall asleep. In my experience, most of my clients go into a deep sleep. Their breathing improves, and fortunately, they are able to eliminate. The staff always thanks me for helping them with elimination. The cues you will use with the client are: "Relax your shoulder and drop your arms and feel like you are holding a penny between your index and thumb area."

Tight shoulders and arms will lead more to chest breathing than diaphragmatic breathing

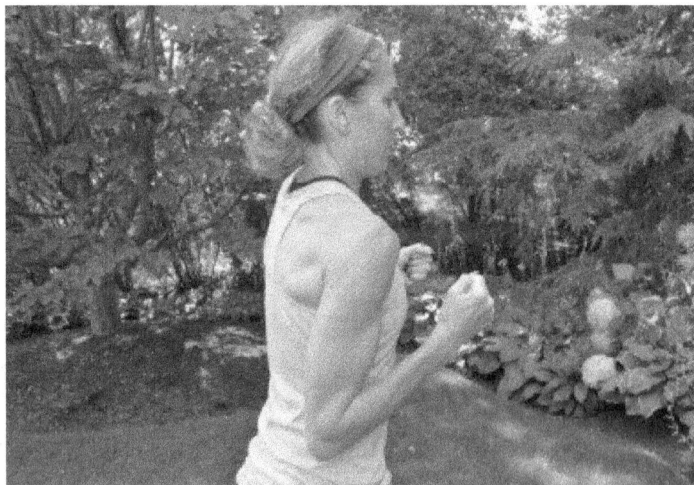

Neurotherapeutic techniques at bicep muscle: holding pressure at bicep muscle and slowly releasing arm into extension

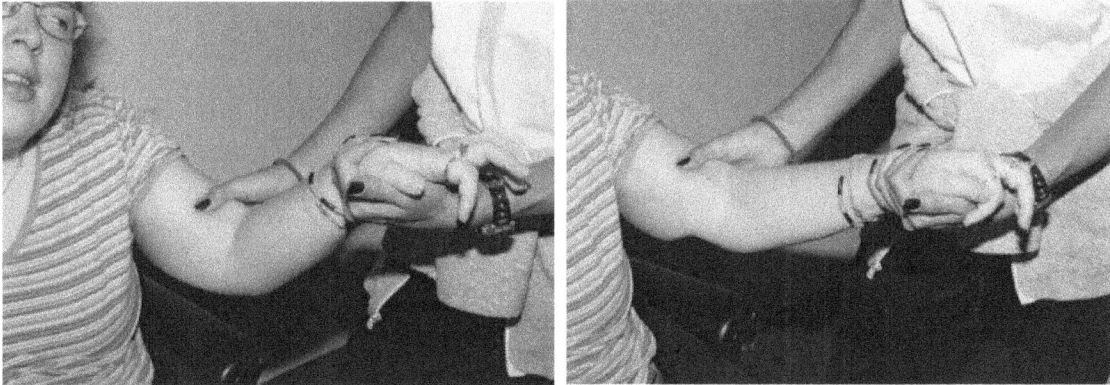

Speaking of shoulders, how many of you know where your shoulder blades are located? Squeezing the shoulder blades together, also known as scapular retraction, can be a difficult task for some people. Bringing the shoulder blades together can automatically bring your head, neck, and back into extension, creating better alignment.

An easy way to teach this concept or correct anatomical positioning is thinking back to the steering wheel example. Place your hands on a make-believe steering wheel. Instead of squeezing the steering wheel with your thumb and your index finger, squeeze your fourth and fifth digits together and then squeeze the steering wheel. What happens to your scapula as you squeeze? Your scapula should retract. Your alignment should improve and your breath should automatically move toward the navel area.

To learn how to squeeze your shoulder blades together so that you can feel the muscles of the scapula contracting, lie supine on your back, with a rolled up towel or a halved piece of foam placed along your spine. From this position, take your fourth and fifth digit and squeeze them together. You should instantly feel your shoulder blades and the muscles around the shoulder blades contracting. Did you feel this?

Scapular retraction using a foam roll and squeezing fourth and fifth digit together

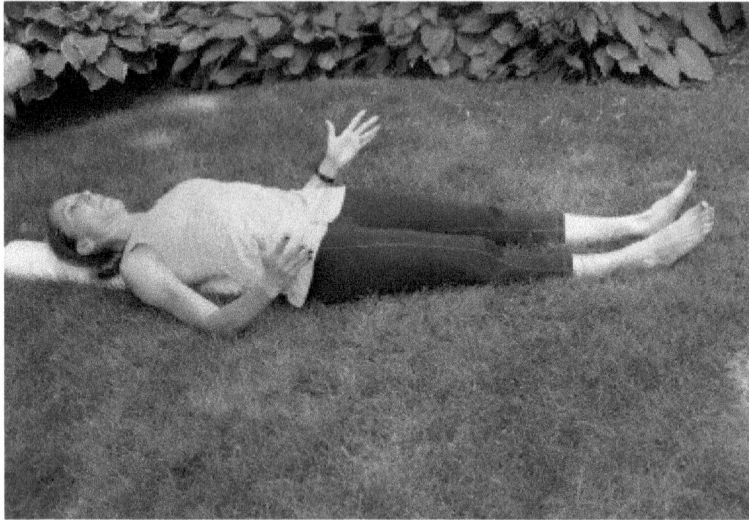

Squeezing fourth and fifth digit to get scapular retraction

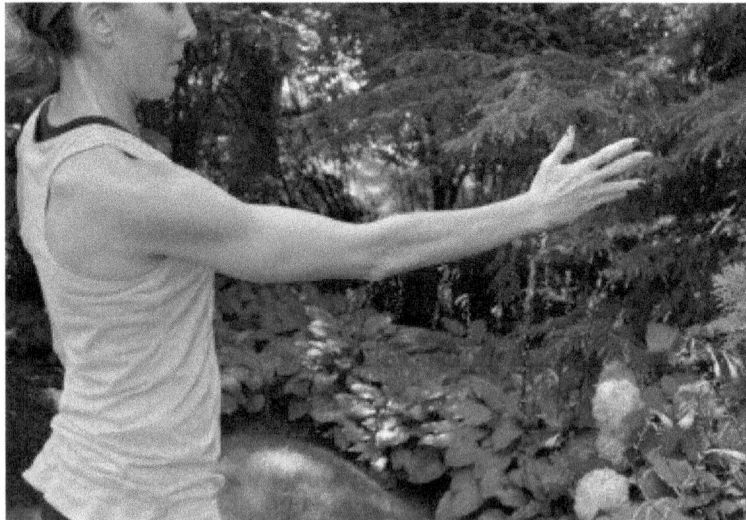

Getting to Know Your Hands and Fingers

I want to share some interesting information about our hands and fingers. In Eastern medicine, the fingers and the hands are considered important areas of the body. In Kundalini yoga, for example, our energy center originates at the navel center and ends up in the palms of the hands and the bottom of the feet. A really strong core will end up circulating oxygen, blood, and energy to the extremities.

Did you know that your fingertips represent different areas of your brain? Researchers have done PET scan studies where simply placing each finger together lights up different areas of the brain. In fact, in Reflexology, it is believed that the total body is reflected in the palm of the hand or the bottom of the foot. You could treat someone's total body by working on the person's hand or foot area.

In my practice working with special needs clients, I have discovered that an easy way to help initiate diaphragmatic breathing if the client is unable to or needs a jump start is to place your thumbs on both palms of the client's hands approximately a one inch below their third, fourth, and fifth digit. Simply apply gentle pressure for about three minutes and watch as the client's diaphragmatic breathing pattern becomes more pronounced. This area corresponds to the same area on the feet so if you would rather hold the feet than the hands, it would result in the same effect.

This procedure also works well with colicky babies, as I discovered when I was on the airplane sitting next to a mom with her baby who had a difficult time settling down. I didn't realize then that I would be working on my own colicky son nine months later.

In Yogic and Buddhists traditions, these hand positions are called mudras. When people meditate, they will often hold their fingers in these different positions or mudras. There are many different types of mudras. Have you ever seen ancient Buddhist or Hindu statues where the hands are sculpted in various positions? These mudras work by putting pressure on meridians in the fingers that affect specific parts of the brain. They hold and direct energy flow and reflexes to the brain.

The most common mudra that you'll see is Gyan Mudra. If the yoga class you attend has already incorporated this mudra, great. If not, Gyan Mudra has a wonderful meaning and you may like to start using it on your own even if it is not used in your class.

In the Gyan Mudra, the index finger touches the thumb. The other three fingers are extended, kind of like an "okay" sign. In fact, when the other three fingers are extended you may try squeezing the fourth and fifth digits together and accomplish good posture with the mudra.

The thumb represents your ego and the index finger actually represents expansion. By performing this mudra, you're actually helping to decrease your ego and reduce your stresses, strains, emotional instabilities, excessive anger, laziness, insomnia, indecisiveness, judgments and negative self-talk. At the same time, you are allowing wisdom, energy, joy, good health and awareness – whatever you desire – to come into your life.

Another well-known mudra is prayer position where the palms of the hands are pressed flat together. You bring the right hand, representing male energy, to the left hand, representing female energy, to help center and balance yourself. Your thumbs actually push on an acupressure point which is known to relieve nervousness, anxiety, chest tension and depression. Now you can understand the power and meaning behind the prayer pose.

Gyan Mudra

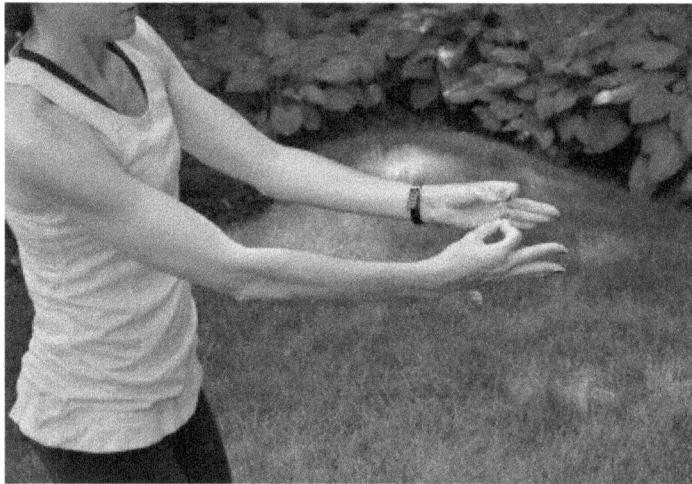

Reflexology Point for the Lungs

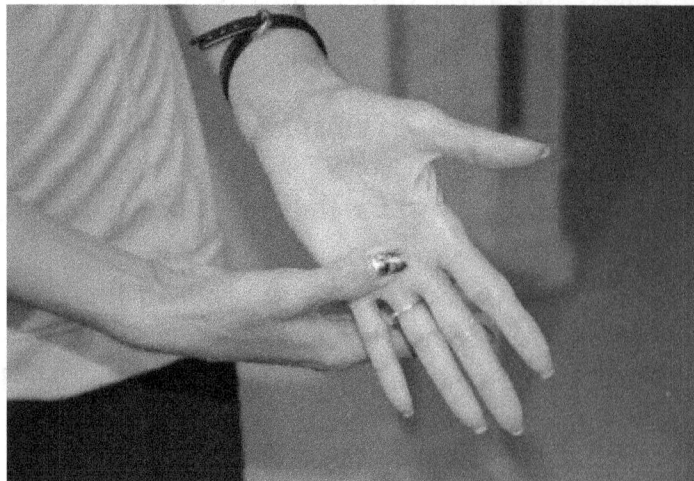

Looking at mudras, Dr. Dharma, author of *Meditation as Medicine,* performed many studies to help individuals improve brain health and prevent Alzheimer's disease, regardless of age and stage of life. He focused his studies on a Kundalini yoga tradition called Kirtan Kriya. This is a simple meditation, using your fine motor skills, your voice, and your ability to go within. Each finger is touched to your thumb, starting with your index finger and ending with your baby finger. The motion is repeated again and again. A mantra is used because sound moves through the connective tissue.

The results of the study were profound. Brain activity improved in areas of the brain central to memory and learning. This area of the brain is known as the hippocampus. Moreover, cognition improved. This meditation also created higher activity in the frontal areas of the brain which are associated with attention, emotions, and memory.

Dr. Dharma's findings on the hippocampus area have led to other research studies focusing on this important gland. Washington University School of Medicine found that school-aged children who were nurtured early in life had brains with a larger hippocampus, the key structure to learning and memory (Luby JL, Barch DM, Belden, A., Gaffey MS, Tillman, R, Babb, C, Nishino T, Suzuki H, and Botteron, KN, 2012).

Let's look at how we can raise our arms upward more easily knowing what you have learned. Reach with your arms up the sky and bring them back down. Don't forget to breathe from the nose keeping your head in neck lock. Drop your jaw, move from the navel center, and hold your hands in the Gyan Mudra, squeezing your fourth and fifth digits. Inhale. Raise your arms up, and exhale, bringing your arms down to your body. If you performed this activity correctly, you probably used good diaphragmatic breathing with good posture and alignment.

Getting to Know Your Eyes

I bet you didn't realize that the eyes have a connection to the breath. The eyes have a great impact on motor skill development, physical body orientation, and protective responses related to peripheral vision.

Go ahead and squeeze them – really tighten your eyes – as if you're having difficulty trying to read a book. My eyes are getting worse as I have aged, and I have noticed that the more squinting I do, the more forward my posture wants to go. As a result, it becomes more challenging for me to breathe, not to mention all the wrinkles that are forming on my forehead from the eye strain and tension.

Now try keeping your eyes wide open without straining and stressing. Do you find your posture in better alignment and your breathing easier?

Did you know we have billions of tiny active units making up the nervous system and they're designed to communicate electrochemically with one another? Each neuron receives and transmits signals through thousands of tiny wires, linking it with other neurons throughout the nervous system (Diagram group, 1983). There are signals going on everywhere within our nervous system, and the brain eventually must be able to take all these signals and interpret them so that we can move and exist. With Nero link Research, it has been found that our bodies contain 100 billion active units, each with 20,000 different connections and that we interpret information from 260 million light receptors in the eyes.

Studies have focused specifically on vision. If you are concentrating on a task and in a hurry, straining your eyes, your breathing pattern will change. It is actually beneficial to be aware of your surroundings, limiting eye strain when performing a task, and keeping your eyes more relaxed and wide open. This will not only not only enhance diaphragmatic breathing, but will also allow you to become more relaxed and connected to the environment around you.

For example, if you are being asked to reach for an item on the table, lessen your direct focus on the item and be aware of other things in the room or on the table so that you become aware of your peripheral surroundings. Try keeping your eyes more open and reach with your scapula pulled back. This will prevent forward reaching and less eye tension. If someone asked you the color of the room and if other items were on the table, you'd be able to answer them successfully.

Why do people close their eyes when they meditate or do yoga? It is because when they close their eyes, it brings them deeply into their body's consciousness. It also centers them into their breath. It focuses them on what is really happening inside.

My clients often come to me have tension and anxiety. The moment I ask them to perform an exercise, guess what? They almost shut down their breathing and go into panic mode. Initially, they may feel that they are being judged. When I ask them to close their eyes and repeat the exercise again, their breath and the fluidity of their movement changes. They feel more secure and relaxed and can actually breathe.

Have you been to a yoga class where they ask you to place your eyes on different areas of your body? In my Kundalini practice, eye focus is a tool.

Here is a simple eye focus exercise to try. Close your eyes and do the best that you can. Keep your eyes closed, and slowly bring them to the third eye point, which is centered between the brows of your eyes. This is where you will activate the pituitary gland and where intuition is developed.

Keep your eyes closed and slowly roll your eyes downward, as if you were looking at your chin. This is a cooling and calming point, and you're going to be able to see yourself more clearly. We call this the moon center.

Keep your eyes closed and roll your eyes to the top of the head or the crown center. This eye focus point will stimulate the pineal gland and the crown energy centers.

These are just a couple of eye focus points that Yogi Bhajan, the master of Kundalini Yoga, shared with the world. Indeed, having a point of focus and closing your eyes will change your breath, posture, and the ability to see yourself more clearly (Bhajan, Y, 2007).

Exploring the Root Lock

The other lock I want to mention, besides neck lock which was mentioned earlier, is the root lock. Any time you are doing an exercise or an activity that requires balance, coordination or control, you will always want to remember to do root lock.

Root lock is a way of squeezing your rectum and your sex organs and bringing your navel towards your spine. It is independent of the breath. It's similar to what we term in women's health as doing Kegel exercises. For men, it helps with the prostate gland. For everyone, this lock will tone the sexual system and move energy up from the lower centers.

Try performing the root lock. As you are squeezing and holding, continue to breathe in and out normally, using conscious breathing. You're securing your pelvis and providing your body with stability and connection to the ground.

Stand up for a moment and remove your shoes. Try balancing yourself on one leg. You can raise one foot and rest it on the lower shin or foot of the other leg. If you feel brave, try the tree pose: bring your heel up to the groin area and stretch your arms overhead with palms together, arms hugging your ears.

Without any conscious preparation, first just try balancing on one leg. Then try balancing on the other. It may be very difficult. Now apply root lock along with neck lock. Relax your jaw and eyes and breathe consciously in and out of your nose. I bet you were able to balance longer and had more stability. What a difference!

Remember doing leg lifts or straight leg raises in gym class? Do you remember if you were using control at your pelvis or were you just lifting your leg up and down in order to complete the required ten repetitions? Do you remember having control over your pelvis and breathing consciously? Do you also realize that when you are performing leg raises that you're actually activating different energy centers of the body?

For example, the straight leg raise exercise is one of the exercises I give to one of my pelvic floor clients. Why? Raising your leg six inches off the ground – the angle used in my yogic practice – has an effect on the ovaries and sex glands. However, as you raise your leg higher like at 90 degrees, your memory and your pineal and pituitary gland will be stimulated.

I would teach my client to perform root lock prior to lifting the leg. Then, as the leg is being raised six inches off the ground, I would coach the client to inhale as the leg is raised and exhale as the leg is lowered, using all the appropriate cues and nasal breathing. By executing this exercise in this manner, you strengthen your pelvis and its surrounding muscles. Your balance and coordination will improve, and you will facilitate a connection in a weakened area.

Getting Acquainted with Standing Up

Stand up and take a moment to feel what it's like to be standing on each leg. You may have to close your eyes to visualize more clearly. Are you leaning or standing on one side or leg more than the other? Most people tend to stand on one leg more dominantly because of habits and functional movement patterns that have not been corrected. Sometimes carrying a backpack on one arm or carrying your baby on one side over the other or just always standing and reaching for things on a shelf using one side versus the other will have an effect on your stance.

Recognize this because the way you are standing is most likely the way you are sitting. Your current stance may also be the reason why you are having issues within your body.

As you are standing there, I'd like you to take a step forward. Did you take a step forward with "your best leg" – the one leg that you are always standing on? Most people usually put their best foot forward.

What has happened with the other leg – the one you didn't move? Are your legs actually imbalanced muscularly or skeletally? Look at the tone of each of your legs? Are you able to see how these patterns of movement can create imbalances all over the body? Perhaps looking in a mirror will help with body clarification. I like to instruct my clients to really lean toward the side they stand on more. What happens is that clients will commonly have to catch their balance to stop themselves from falling toward that strong stance side. This cue is vital to bringing awareness to a repetitive movement pattern that will require modification (Bond, M, 2007).

Trying Indian sitting or Easy Pose Versus W Sitting

Take a moment to sit on the ground with your legs crisscrossed in what is called Indian sitting or Easy Pose. If you noticed a stronger stance side from the experiment that you just performed, now when you are sitting, are you still leaning toward that same side? Are you repeating this movement pattern with other postures? Are you sitting straight with a neutral spine or are you leaning forward, compressing your diaphragm? You may need to position a pillow under your buttocks to bring your spine, head and neck straight so you can breathe better.

Try sitting in W-sitting position with your knees adducted or pressing together. This means sitting on your bottom on the floor with your knees bent and rotated so that they are touching the floor in the shape of a "W". Lots of kids like to sit in this position. It definitely is not a recommended position. This position can cause problems with stability in the trunk and hips, orthopedic issues with the hips, knees, and feet, tightness in the hamstrings, hip adductors, and heel cords, and decreased trunk rotation. The core connection to the diaphragm gets closed with this position, making breathing more difficult. Take a moment and try conscious, nasal breathing in this position. I guarantee that you are breathing more from your chest than your diaphragm.

Now stand up and bring your knees together almost like a standing "W" position. Try breathing through the nose and observe if your breathing also feels challenged.

Tom Meyers, in his book *Anatomy Trains*, gives us some insights as to why this position is so negative. Meyers has played an integral role in fascial mapping. His knowledge and study of the body has made it easier for us today to truly understand how the body is connected.

He describes the deep front line or core line. Some of the muscles or structures involved are the cranium and facial bones, the jaw muscles, the diaphragm, the multifidi, the psoas, pelvis area, lesser trochanter of femur (hip bone), adductor brevis and longus and adductor magnus (muscles in the middle of your thighs), medial femoral epicondyle (bone on inside of knee joint) ,posterior tibia/fibula (bones on back of lower limbs), and plantar tarsal bones (bone on bottom of feet) and the plantar surface of the toes (area on bottom of feet) . This deep front line helps lift up the inner arch, supports the lumbar spine from the front, balances our head and neck, helps with breathing, and stabilizes each segment of the legs. This line enhances our breathing, the rhythm of our walking, and the stabilization of our head and neck. (Myers, T, 2006). Because closing off your knees through adduction in W sitting or standing will close down this integral fascial chain and disrupt the core line, this posture leads to poor breathing, poor rhythmic walking, and problems with head and neck stabilization.

W-sitting

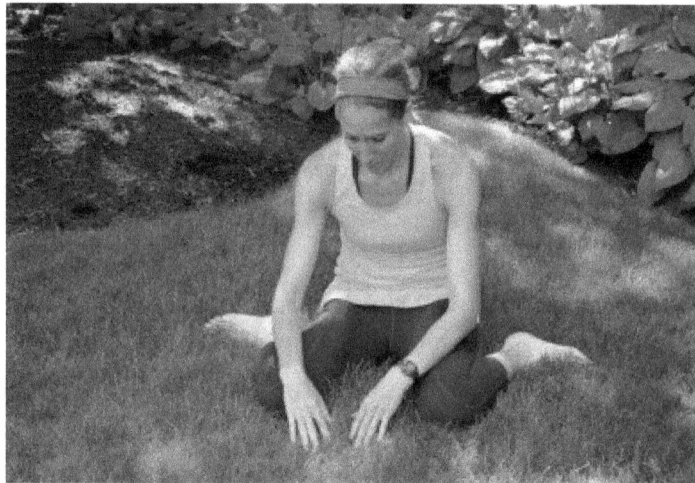

Exploring Your Arches

When your foot hits the ground, it translates motion all the way to the top of your head. We tend to stand on what we call our functional center of the foot, which is our tarsal sinus (Bond, M, 2007).Our tarsal sinus is located directly in front of the lateral malleolus, the bony prominence on each side of the ankle. Or if you draw a line from the fourth toe, the tarsal sinus is in that little groove.

When we pronate or when we supinate our foot, that little dimple should get bigger or smaller. Most people kind of hang out on their tarsal sinus. As a result, their arches collapse or they pronate which is the inward roll of your foot during normal motion.

Stand up now and pronate your feet (roll them inward), and try to breathe diaphragmatically. Is it difficult? Now supinate your feet or roll them outward, and breathe. Was that easier?

If you are standing on a collapsed arch, you're shutting down this deep line connection. Remember, I just mentioned this core connection between the diaphragm, the pelvic floor, the transverse abdominis, the lumbar multifidi, the jaw, the adductor magnus, and all the way down to the plantar muscles and to the medial arch. As you can see, a dropped arch can result in TMJ issues.

Our body attempts to tells us the truth when we are sick or healthy, but sometimes the symptoms can be hard to interpret. For instance, a person might have a sore elbow, but the problem might be a displaced rib in the back. You can't always guess the cause from where the pain is located. It is important to remember, however, that our bodies give us signals and to be aware of these signals.

When we walk, upon the heel strike, our foot naturally moves into slight pronation. Then, upon toe off, our foot goes into supination. It is important to know that too much of one of these movements can cause imbalances anywhere along the fascial chain.

Locating Tarsal Sinus

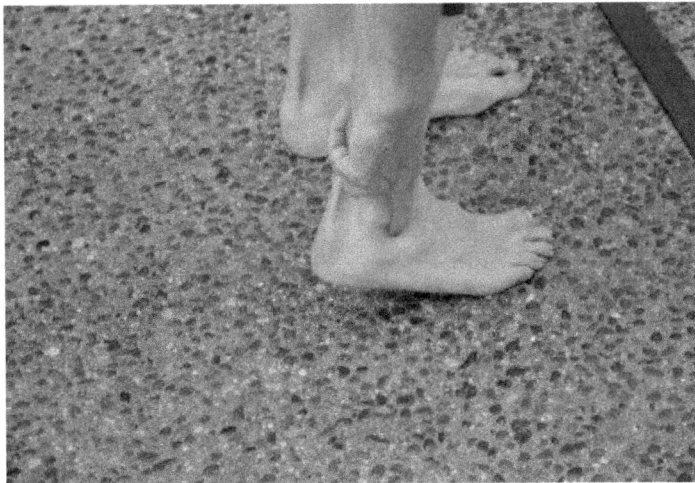

W" position in standing, knees turned in and adducted arches collapsed

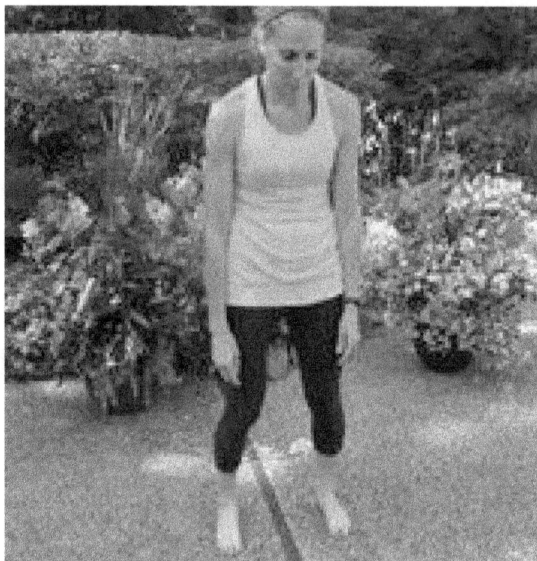

Exploring Your Walking

The standing/walking test requires walking along a straight line, similar to a sobriety test. What I look for with this test is arm swing, equal weigh bearing, and rhythm during walking. I also observe if there is equal space between the arms, overall posture and alignment, head rotation and position, and pelvic alignment.

Addressing pelvic alignment is always the first step in any self-correction exercise. Let me share with you an example about one of my clients who had body awareness issues and required movement and awareness retraining. Her name, whom I'll call Dee, and she came to see me because she was fed up with therapy. She was desperately looking for someone who could help cure her problem. She presented her case to me and claimed that her left knee pain would not go away, even after she had recent surgery on it and had gone through months of rehabilitation. Dee went on to tell me that she had surgery on her right foot ten years previously.

I initially looked at her posture and the fascia on her face which made it clear to me what was wrong. I had her stand up against a wall and evaluated her, visualizing a straight line going through the middle of her body from the top of her head to the bottom of her feet. She was standing more on her right leg than her left leg. Her head position, the distance between her arms, her pelvic alignment, and her shoulder positioning were all off balance.

Dee presented with her head side bent to the right and rotated to the left. The fascia was pulling on the right side of her face, giving me clues of a right-sided issue. Around the umbilicus area, the tissue was pulling down on the right toward the psoas muscle. She stood bearing more weight on her right side with her pelvis rotated to the right. Her right shoulder was lower than her left shoulder and the space between her arms was greater on the left than on the right.

I asked her why she thought she had knee pain, but she had no idea. I asked her to walk a straight line which I had clearly marked with masking tape. Just as I thought, she leaned so much to the right that her right foot crossed the tape. Her left foot had to stabilize and control her entire body to prevent her from falling to the right. The left side of her body was overstressed and taking a lot of pressure. She even displayed little ankle mobility and heel toe strike on the right foot, meaning she spent most of her time with her right foot pronated on the ground.

The cause of her problem was poor ankle mobility from a surgery ten years ago which had affected her fascial chain. The left knee problem was due to over compensation issues. Her left knee pain would not disappear until she connected with and became aware of her habitual posture. The pull of her body to the right was throwing off her gravitational line, leading to balance and coordination problems. Interestingly, her right foot was making a loud tapping noise when it hit the ground and her left foot hardly made any noise.

My treatment plan for her encompassed increasing her awareness of her body by postural corrections in the mirror; range of motion and joint mobilization exercises for her right foot; muscle stretching for the right side and strengthening for left side of her body; and gait training with postural corrections using the standing/walking test and breath walk exercises. Due to the poor diaphragmatic breathing caused by her poor posture and alignment, I also included breathing exercises in supine, sitting, and standing positions. Postural alignment involved aligning her pelvis first; then her shoulders; correcting her head positioning and then her stance. Her left knee wasn't the initial problem after all, but the true cause of all her instabilities and pains arose from immobility within her right ankle.

Let me add that sound or rhythm is important with the deep frontal line. A lot of my clients are visually impaired, so they have to rely on their auditory system to get proprioceptive feedback. This auditory feedback – listening to her footsteps – helped Dee realize when she was walking more on her right foot than her left foot. She closed her eyes, listened to her walking pattern and received that immediate feedback. I helped her create music and rhythm within her gait pattern. These were combined with visual and tactile cueing, so that she would actually start to breathe, open up and walk in alignment again. Dee had to learn to develop a heel-toe gait pattern again. It was using the breath walk, a form of walking where you link the rhythm of your breath with your step that helped Dee increase the energy to her system, boost her circulation, and reconnect and rebalance her body.

Did you know that you can learn to increase your inhalations and exhalations by performing more steps? Try inhaling for two steps instead of one and then exhaling for three steps. Remember the postural cues: head in neck lock; jaw relaxed; eyes relaxed; squeeze your fourth and fifth digit; relax your shoulders and move from the navel center.

Standing Straight line Walking Test

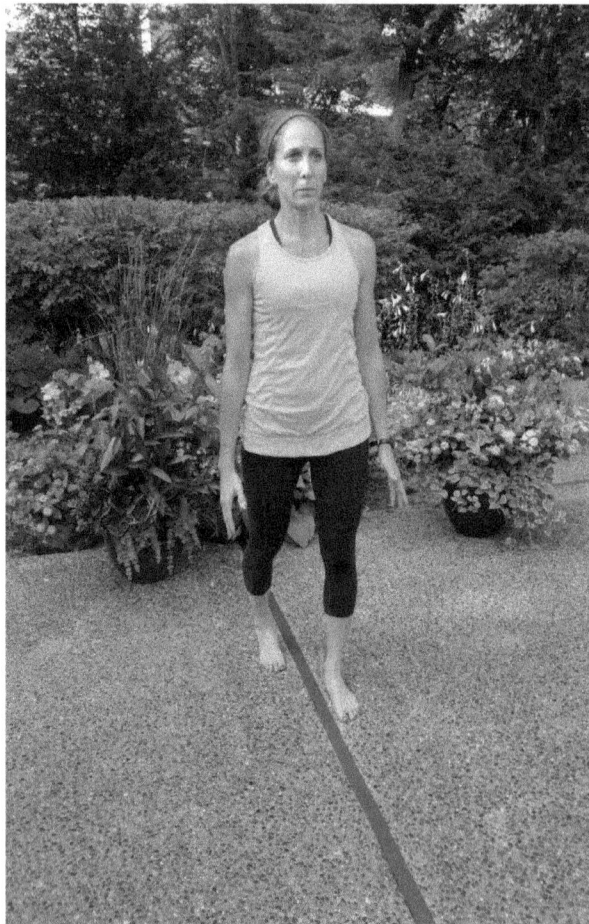

Example of how Dee was walking during standing walking test

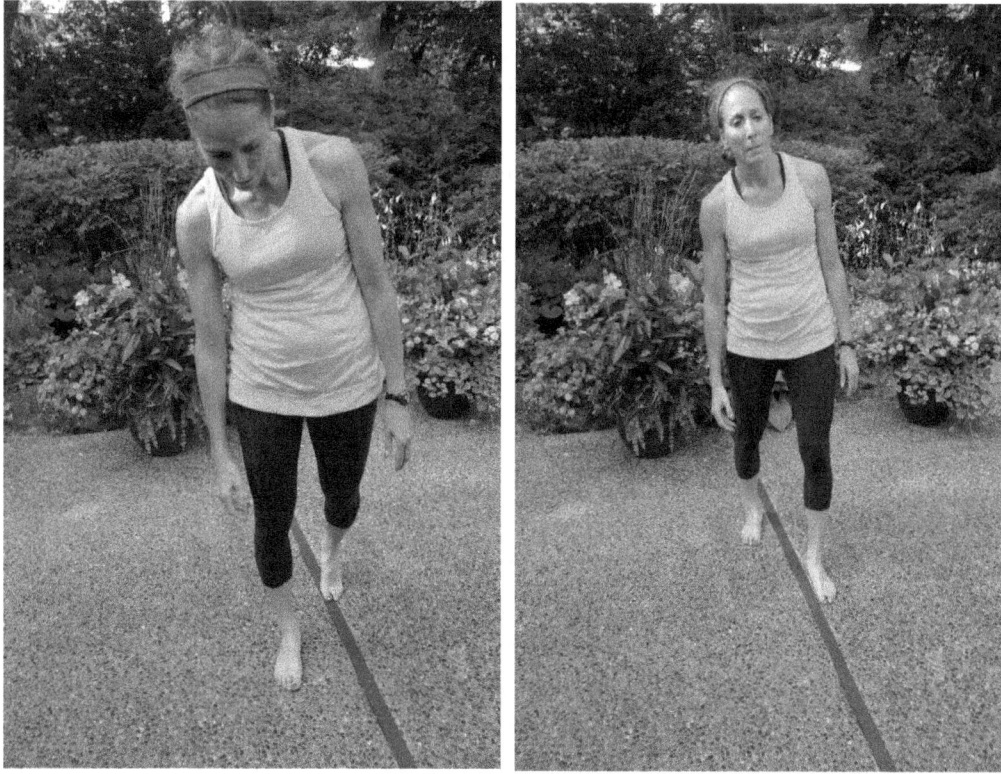

Exploring Sound

Sound is a sensory component used in breath walk. The ears are the first things to develop within the womb. Sound travels four times faster in water. The body is about 70 percent water, which makes the body a perfect resonator for sound. Our bones and our bone marrow have high water content. Sound therefore connects with the bone marrow and the stem cells and will also affect cellular regeneration.

Dr. Alfred Tomatis, a French Ear, Nose, and Throat Specialist, found that all the cranial nerves lead to the ear. He showed that the ear is neurologically involved with the optic and ocular motor nerves; therefore, it is interrelated with vision and movement. It is also related to the vagus nerve or cranial nerve number ten which affects the larynx, the bronchi, the heart, and the GI tract. Thus, the ear affects our voice, our breathing, our heart rate, and our digestion. Sound moves through our connective tissue helping with fascial pathway corrections (Bond, M., 2007).

Sound has been used for years in therapy. Drumming in the early 70's was used to help with endorphin release. There is research on using music with children with autism, and they found these children could understand and connect better with people using music or sound therapy. I have personally helped clients, either those who have had a stroke or young children who are developmentally delayed, to learn how to talk again. They place their hands on my vocal cords to feel the vibration of the word they want to speak. They then vibrate or sing the sound or word back to me.

Human hearing ranges from 20 to 20,000 hertz, depending upon age and health of the person. In my profession, ultrasound is used, which is basically utilizing a sound crystal to help move energy through the system. A dolphin or whale can hear up to frequencies of 50,000 hertz. How many of you ever heard of dolphin therapy before? Dolphin therapy exists in California, Florida, and Puerto Vallarta. Dolphins can emit higher frequency sound wavelengths, helping to cure and treat certain diseases more effectively than our standard ultrasound machines. Sound is, indeed, therapeutic.

The real reason why people chant or use sound therapy is because vibrating the 84 meridians or channels located on the hard palate and the soft palate helps open up the pathway to the hypothalamus, the pituitary gland, and the pineal gland. This form of stimulation is a perfect way to not only secrete endorphins throughout your system but also release powerful hormones and glands for ultimate health. It is very simple to do. Just say words where your tongue hits the hard and soft palate, like Namaste, friend or rabbit, and you will open up channels for these hormones and endorphins and be in bliss.

Exploring Visual Deficits

How many of you are visual learners? How many of you teach through the visual system? The majority of the population today teaches through visual learning. What happens if the visual system is impaired? You will have to teach through another modality, most commonly the auditory system. Sometimes you will have to go to a kinesthetic approach if the person has both visual and auditory impairments.

Visual issues exist within our society. Children in school today who have social and behavioral problems may have visual deficits. Children with minimal brain dysfunction and even criminals in the jail system have been known to have visual deficits. Effects of neurological insults on vision can include: reduced focusing, strabismus or misalignment of the eyes, instability or postural changes, tracking problems, vestibular effects on eye movement, visual field loss, abnormal light sensitivity, visual perception issues, and reduced blinking rate. These neurological insults on vision can affect ambulation, hand-eye coordination, perception, cognition, depth perception, self-feeding, reading, balance, and driving (Chaikin, Laurie, 2013).

Some children with autism are known to be toe walkers. Why toe walking? Alan Kaplan, in his book, *Seeing through New Eyes: Changing the Lives of Children with Autism, Asperger Syndrome, and Developmental Disorders through Vision Therapy,* reports that the majority of us have what is called good focal vision. Meaning that if I point to an object, like a glass, and ask you what it is, you would say, "It's a glass."

Now, let's pretend that I'm going to throw a ball to you. You know it is a ball, but the moment that I throw the ball, you quickly turn away or look in a different direction. This is called ambient vision, meaning you can't process all the sensory information coming to you from the outside world or from the environment. You would have poor spatial reasoning and would have difficulty recognizing where the object is coming from in space.

Researchers are finding that children with autism have really good focal vision, but they have poor ambient vision. For example if you are on a plane and there was turbulence on the plane, what would you do with your feet? You would most probably do what? Put them flat on the ground, right? What would you do with your toes? Kind of grip the ground, right? What's happens with autistic children is that they don't know where they're moving in space, so they're performing the way that their bodies are responding. They're gripping the ground. And they're toe walking, because they don't feel secure in their space.

People ask, 'Why don't they become heel walkers?" If you had a visual issue, what would you want to do with your eyes? The most secure place is where? Of course, it's the ground. So these children walk looking at the ground, their toes are gripping the ground, and their posture is going forward. They are trying to find their way around in space. If they became heel walkers, their head and neck would become extended and their eyes would be looking up to the sky, lacking any connection to the world around them.

Did you know that most schools within the United States are actually required to execute visual screening tests? However, most schools and some eye doctors only test for visual acuity and not for other visual problems.

Do you know that when you go to the eye doctor they mainly test for visual acuity, being able to sit or stand 20 feet away and read the letters on a chart? I'm sure you know this test well if you have ever gone to an eye doctor. Are your eyes moving or doing anything?

A good doctor would have you read the letters in all different planes of motion, reading the chart diagonally, horizontally, backwards – every possible way – because our eyes would have to track in all planes, just as if you were reading a book. Other specialized vision tests, unfortunately, aren't performed at most eye doctor visits. Some of these tests can verify a true visual deficit, like an eye muscle test and a range of motion of the eyes, tests for double vision, visual perception tests, and even tests for strabismus. A classroom vision checklist, such as the one I use, may include appearance of the eyes, complaints when using eyes at the desk, behavioral signs of visual deficits, eye teaming abilities, eye hand coordination issues, and visual form perception issues.

Dr. John Downing in 2009 discovered different pathways of light. His knowledge has helped us understand the vision system better. It is known that when light hits the eye, it goes through the thalamus, the sensory relay station. From there, it travels to the visual cortex and then it makes its way either to the limbic system, the part of the brain that controls our emotions, or to the cerebral cortex of the brain, responsible for most high brain functions such as language, memory, and consciousness. Finally, it passes on to other areas of the brain.

Dr. Downing found two unique direct pathways of light. The first pathway is that when light hits the eye it can go directly to the brainstem, the part of our brain responsible for coordination, balance, posture, respiration, and stability. Clients who have balance and coordination issues are now using balanced-torso weighted vests to not only help with balance and coordination issues, but also to retrain their visual system which is the main culprit causing their instability.

The second direct pathway discovered is linked to the endocrine system and many of our other anatomical systems. With this pathway, when light hits the eye, it either goes directly to the hypothalamus, to the pituitary gland, the thyroid gland, and even to our adrenal glands or it goes from the hypothalamus directly to the pineal gland. It is now known that autonomic nervous system dysfunction – as well as endocrine dysfunction – may stem from visual field deficits. Correcting visual deficits can help to balance the entire nervous system – both the autonomic nervous system, and all other systems connected.

I'd like to just give you a brief neuroanatomy overview. The hypothalamus is a tiny organ responsible for regulating our breathing, heart rate, blood pressure, thirst, and our sweat. It is not only an endocrine organ, but it also is part of the nervous system. It regulates and remains under involuntary control when the autonomic nervous system is under stress. It is responsible for overseeing both the parasympathetic and sympathetic branch of the autonomic nervous system.

If the body has too much stress and trauma, the hypothalamus can't stay balanced, thus throwing off the entire glandular system. That creates imbalance throughout our bodies.

That is why we begin aging in our twenties. Our emotional state of mind, governed by the amygdala, an endocrine organ, causes the hypothalamus to evaluate every situation. If our emotional state becomes unstable, then it will have a direct effect on our pituitary gland and on our hippocampus, the endocrine gland responsible for learning and memory.

The pituitary gland, one of the glands that may have problems if the hypothalamus isn't functioning correctly, is considered a major gland for secretion of three major hormones: thyroid, adrenal, and reproductive. It supports bone maturation, milk production, bone synthesis, protein synthesis and the use of our fat reserves. It contains magnetite, iron, and oxygen, which may explain our sensitivity to magnetic fields (Dale, Cindy, 2009).

The thyroid gland, on the other hand, releases thyroid hormone which controls the speed of the body's chemical functions and regulates our basal metabolic function, which aids in the beating of our heart, respiration and maintenance of our body temperature. The adrenal glands are located on top of the kidneys and have two parts: the cortex and the medulla. The cortex produces cortisol, an anti-inflammatory hormone that converts protein to energy and releases stored sugar so our bodies have enough fuel to respond as needed. The medulla, the inner part, secretes epinephrine, also called adrenaline, and norepinephrine. Both are involved in the stress response, and are linked to the nervous system, respiratory system, and circulatory system. Breath alone can quite clearly govern and help regulate these endocrine glands.

Did you know that the optic nerve lies between the hypothalamus and the pituitary gland? It is easy now to see that when light hits the eye it will have a direct effect on these two organs.

The pituitary gland lies just behind our brow point. Stroking this point, as my mom did when I was a baby to put me to sleep at night, or bowing and touching your forehead, the brow point, on the ground, can activate the pituitary gland, along with the hypothalamus and optic nerve area.

Dr. Downing found that when light hits the eye, it will go through the hypothalamus and to the pineal gland. The pineal gland is under study today. It produces a hormone called melatonin which affects a lot of our life force, our DHEA, and our human growth hormone. Melatonin is greatly responsible for our sleep/wake cycle. When we age, the majority of us sleep less. As we lose sleep, our melatonin levels go down, which will then affect the whole balancing of our hypothalamus. Yogis and the people in the Eastern world get up early in the morning - before the sun rises – because they actually found that there is a shift in hormone levels. It actually transforms from melatonin to norepinephrine, epinephrine, and cortisol naturally.

I am not only a writer, but I do a lot of public speaking. One thing I love about being a speaker is that when I ask the Universe to supply me with information, I'm often guided to the source or location of this information. I was in a book store and was guided to a book titled: *Under the Weather: How the Weather and Climate Affect our Health* by Pat Thomas. It was very synchronistic.

The book discusses all the weather changes that our occurring within our world and how these changes can increase our risk for health issues. I laugh because I live in Phoenix, Arizona. As I write this, it is summer and it is hot, 116 degrees. I'm watching outside my window as a dust storm called a haboob is approaching. These dark, dusty storms make visibility dangerous. You wouldn't want to be driving in one of these storms. Haboobs are apparently becoming more frequent these days. I wonder what these haboobs are doing to our health. In fact, this book mentions that when there are a lot of solar flares, heart attack rates increase.

I opened the book and there was a description about the pineal gland:

> "It's sometimes referred to as a third eye, and believed to be the seat of the human soul. The pineal gland is exquisitely sensitive to its surroundings, and acts as a mediator between man and his environment. In response to light and darkness, it secretes the hormone melatonin, which is widely understood to be responsible for our sleep/wake cycles. But it's also involved in regulating growth and mental stability. Low levels of this important hormone have been implicated in modern health problems, such as cancer, hypertension, and sexual dysfunction. Malfunctions of the pineal gland have also been linked to epilepsy, schizophrenia, and autism"(Thomas, P. 2004).

This little gland mediates the production of nitric-oxide, a chemical that helps to regulate our breathing. In my practice of Kundalini yoga, Yogi Bhajan believed that after the eighth year in life, the pineal gland does not secrete fully and that it acquires the reserve energy stored at the navel point. Reaching universal awareness requires an unwinding of the energy, moving it from the navel center and connecting it with the pineal gland. That's again why this core connection is important. It is because the more we are connected at the navel center, the higher our melatonin levels will be.

As a physical therapist, when it's a full moon I know that my day of work will be quite interesting. My clients with epilepsy or seizure disorder are likely to have seizures during that day, and my other clients may display unusual behaviors. The term lunatic literally means "moon sick".

Seizure disorder is an abnormal electrical activity of the brain. Think about it. During the full moon, it is light outside all night long. When it is dark outside, we are used to sleeping and our bodies are naturally producing melatonin. When it is a full moon, because it stays light outside all night long, our bodies sleep/wake cycle gets thrown off. Clients who have seizures are more than likely to have increased seizure activity during this time. I felt this personally when I was in Alaska during the summer when there was nearly twenty-four hours of daylight. It made me a little crazy. I didn't know if it was day or night or even what day it was.

In the 1920's, Dr. Spitler theorized the role of the eyes in photo transduction and the role of light and color in biological function and development. He believed many dysfunctions were caused by imbalances in the autonomic nervous system and endocrine system. He spoke about the retinal-hypothalamic-pituitary axis. He proposed that applying certain frequencies of light through the eyes could create balance and correct visual dysfunctions at their source.

Exploring the Effects of Color

As early as 1697, Isaac Newton looked at color through a prism and said that individual colors have a certain frequencies or vibrations to them. Dr. Spitler used color to help with the nervous and endocrine system. Dr. Spitler looked at three major colors: red, blue, and yellow. He used red to help with sympathetic nervous system dysfunctions and blue to help activate the parasympathetic nervous system. Yellow was used as a visual stimulant. His work led me and others to use color for treatment purposes.

I have done much work with clients who had incomplete spinal cord injuries. I'd wrap a red sheet or a towel around the affected body parts to activate them, helping to work subconsciously and involuntarily through the autonomic nervous system. Using red in treatment can indeed enhance mobility. Wearing red lenses can help increase your muscle tone and strength, alleviate depression, improve alertness, increase your energy, and bring your posture more into extension (change your postural perspective), making you feel more upright. Your breath will even shift.

Look at all the colors that are used for marketing. Red is a what – an appetite stimulant? Why are so many restaurants today painted red? It's because they are trying to get you to eat their food and, of course, spend money. Never paint your kitchen red or you might find yourself gaining weight. I also recommend that you never paint your bedroom the color red and avoid using red sheets because you might find yourself with insomnia caused by overstimulation.

After taking my course, a classroom teacher discovered why one of her autistic students couldn't sit still on Fridays. Fridays were school color day and guess what the school color was? RED! Red is powerful and if you have a hard time focusing and sitting, this probably wouldn't be the best color choice for you.

On the other hand, for those of you who live in cold climates, depression may set it. You can sit cure your depression by wearing red lenses. It will give you a different perspective on life. My son's favorite color is red. He is such a high energy child. As a mom I'm thinking about changing his wardrobe to blue clothes and limit the amount of red toys.

Animals are also really sensitive to color. Let me share a quick story. I was in Thailand at a monastery, a wildlife refuge, and was able to walk along the enclosure for the lions and the tigers. Of course, I was under the direction of the monks who took care of the animals. I remember the day clearly. I was wearing an orange shirt with red flowers. I walked into the monastery, and the monk in charge looked at me, and he said, "You can't go in there."

I said, "Why can't I go in there?"

And he said, "Because you're going to scare the animals. It's your shirt! Didn't you read the book?"

I replied, "No, I didn't read the book. I'm on vacation."

He handed me a black shirt and told me to put it on. He then informed me that the color red will really affect the animals and make them frightened.

Blue, on the other hand, is calming and relaxing. I often want to teach my lectures wearing blue lenses. Blue assists me become grounded within my body. Blue helps decrease anxiety, relaxes your muscles and body, and makes your posture more relaxed. You may know people with COPD, emphysema, asthma, or clients who hyperventilate. When you are afraid to breathe, wearing blue lenses can help.

There's an interesting study with Helen Irlen. She did research on visual dysfunction of children within the schools. She started using blue transparencies over white worksheets for these children with visual dysfunction because it would actually relax their eyes. They could focus and could see the letter better on blue than on a white background.

Yellow is a really good visual stimulant. I've worked alongside vision therapists who use yellow for clients with visual dysfunction because you can see shadows with the color yellow. I now incorporate the color yellow everywhere in treatment. I use yellow plates, yellow spoons, yellow tape for mobility and yellow balls, etcetera. There is truth to the saying, "Follow the yellow-brick road?" Why did they make McDonalds sign the color yellow? Why are they making yellow legal pads today? Why, after cataract surgery, are they using yellow lenses for recovering patients? Why do people who have night blindness wear yellow lenses? Yellow makes the visual field more pronounced and assists to regulate all those other areas – the hypothalamus, the pituitary gland, and the pineal gland.

Those of you who work with pediatrics or have had children, do you know why tummy time, placing a baby on his/her stomach while awake or supervised, is so important? Yes, we do want our children to develop good extension throughout their trunk and neck area. But, the real reason that we put our children prone is because we want to work on their visual field at a young age.

Judy Jennings in 2008 did research on tummy time for infants. She said that the critical period of peak plasticity for visual acuity and visual perception, being able to see and give meaning to any visual information that encircles us, is under one year of age. This makes clear to us the importance of developing our vision at a very young age. Let me reiterate that science is finding that children today who have learning disabilities or have social problems may also have some type of visual deficit. So it's important that we really evaluate vision early on.

A Case Study

I'd like to share a case study with you. It is difficult sometimes to teach clients with special needs how to breathe properly. One of my clients whom I'll call David is 30-years-old and diagnosed with Cerebral Palsy. He is a highly intelligent young man who is a mouth breather and has some visual deficits. He has high tone throughout his upper and lower extremities, causing him to sit in a very forward flexed posture, knees to chest, and legs adducted or crossed. He uses his eyes and some sounds to communicate with me.

David presents with problems with diaphragmatic breathing, poor body connection, and decreased mobility. I asked him his goals and he always looked toward this walker, called a Meywalker. I explained to him that that was a great goal, realizing that he hadn't waked since he was in his teens and now he is in his forties.

Treatment included placing him on the mat on his back to work on neurotherapeutic techniques to decrease his tone, breathing exercises, body awareness, pressure points to assist with diaphragmatic breathing, wearing blue glasses to relax his tone, and most importantly, having him reconnect with his body using sensory integration. I became the messenger to help him, but David did all the work.

In order for his tone to decrease, he had to learn how to control it. In the past, David was in the hospital for a lot for chronic constipation and respiratory issues. I wondered why.

During the eight months we worked together, his breathing pattern changed and his mobility improved. He learned how to relax and move with decreased tone. He had better circulation, a better attitude, and improved respiration and circulation as verified by less illness and less hospitalizations. The only real weaknesses was having him learn how to reduce outside stimulation for better body concentration and needing at times verbal follow through with staff.

The good news is David eventually was able to walk again. When I placed him in the walker, it was humorous because he apparently had a lot of things to say to people. He would walk almost into these people as though telling them, "See I can do it!" David was grateful and gave me lots of thanks. I told him to not thank me but to thank himself because he did all the work.

In the May 2014 *PT in Motion* magazine, "Making Core Connections," physical therapist Julie Wiebe contributed her thoughts about the importance of the breath. Her findings are very appropriate to summarize this chapter of this book. She used a clinical approach and used "breath as a gateway to activate the central stability system for patients seeking help with balance issues, low-back and hip pain, and poor frontal plane control that leads to knee injuries". So it is now clear that posture, vision, and the breath are linked.

Chapter 8: Research Supporting the Benefits of Proper Ventilation in Disease Prevention

"Realize that everything connects to everything else."
Leonardo da Vinci

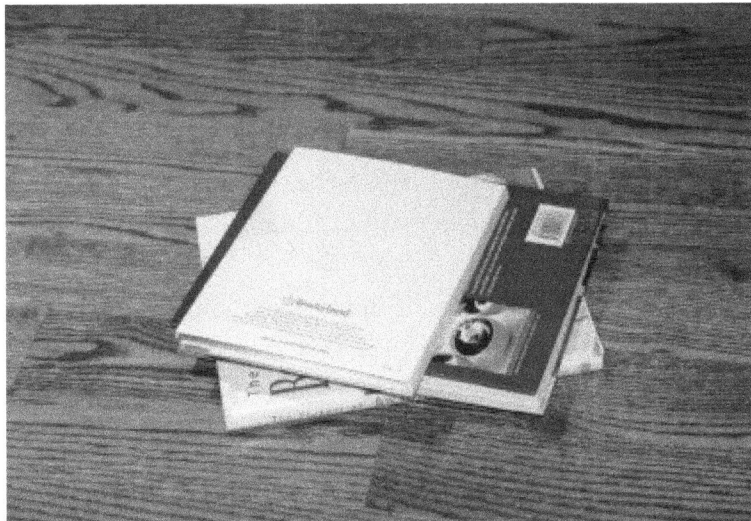

Research helps us to study and investigate new ideas in order to establish facts and generate conclusions. Many studies out there today confirm the importance of breath and demonstrate how our body and all of its systems are connected.

An interesting article titled "The Body of Thought" by Siri Carpenter was presented to me by my son's preschool teacher. This article explains how research is discovering that our higher cognitive processes – our minds – are grounded in our body experiences and in the neuro-circuitry that controls the body (Carpenter, Siri, 2011).

Other research shows that our bodies can't lie. The body is the controller of the mind for knowledge. It is the collector of all our information from our senses. We can truly understand our emotions and how we act by looking to our bodies and not our minds first and foremost. However, our mind may sometimes give the body inaccurate information or interpret the body's responses incorrectly. For instance, your body may say it's tired or sleepy, an emotion, but it may really be dehydrated. It is important to really focus in on what the body is telling us and know that for the majority of the time, we can trust in the innate wisdom of the body.

Our mind sometimes is the culprit which prevents our bodies from doing what they know to do. There were multiple studies cited within "The Body of Thought" to explain this concept. For example, the researchers had a person hold a cup of coffee versus a can of coke. What happened to the person's body when it held the cup of coffee? The body already knew what to do before the mind even thought that it was a cup of coffee. Of course, the person's body relaxed when holding the cup of coffee making him/her feel more warmly toward the people around him/her. On the other hand, the person with the can of coke became more anxious.

Next, they examined undergraduates to see if they would end up being good negotiators. They used a chair in this experiment. Those who sat in hard chairs automatically displayed the body posturing of a good negotiator. Those who sat in soft chairs reacted differently. Their posture was more relaxed, lacking a good negotiator's posture.

The article also mentions what happens with Botox injections. I thought this was humorous. An injection of Botox can jam the neural circuits responsible for processing emotions. Woman or men who decide to have Botox treatments may soon realize that it becomes really hard for their body to recognize emotions when their face is so tight and immoveable.

Another study in this article looked at a person's response when certain words were spoken through headphones. The idea was that once the person heard the word, his/her hand needed to be raised. The results showed that the person's left hand was raised when words about the past were heard, and when the words sounded like the future, the person automatically raised his/her right hand. The body knew that the right hand or side of the body represented the future or forward movement and the left side represented the past.

The Journal of Neurological Research, March of 1999, cited a study in which children scored higher in math tests after taking piano lessons. This discovery was named the Mozart effect, which is a technique of using music to teach spatial and temporal reasoning. Because they are using their fingers constantly, musicians are continuously stimulating different areas of the brain all the time. Remember the mudras? This is the same principle. (Shaw, Gordan, 1999)

How many of you are parents who worry that computers aren't very good for your child's development? Are iPods really beneficial? Surprisingly, Siri Carpenter describes the work of Arthur Glenberg and his colleagues which showed that the best way for children to learn to read and to improve their reading comprehension is not just by sitting there and reading, but by actually doing physical manipulations with their hands. By physically manipulating toys or manipulating images of toys on a computer screen, children were learning how to read faster, and their reading comprehension was actually better than if they were just pointing and reading a book (Carpenter, Siri, 2011). Our fingertips and our brain centers are guiding us into becoming better readers and learners. Our body has all the answers.

How many of you do craniosacral and myofascial work? In addition to our visual system being important for sensory processing, there is now research that points out that our richest and largest sensory organ is not the eyes, ears, skin, or vestibular system, but it is, in fact, our muscles with their related fascia. The connective tissue is a doorway to activating the autonomic nervous system.

One can see why this is so by looking at a typical motor nerve. Three-fourths of that motor nerve is innervated by sensory fibers rather than motor fibers. There are many types of sensory fibers. Golgi fibers help decrease tone. Pacini fibers are used as proprioceptive feedback for movement control. The interstitial type three and four fibers are the most abundant receptor types and are found almost everywhere, even inside of the bones. These type three and four fibers have a direct connection to the autonomic nervous system.

As you are doing tissue manipulation, cranial sacral work, or myofascial work within the connective tissue, you instantly stimulate these mechanoreceptors, which trigger the autonomic nervous system. As a result, the local fluid dynamics within the tissue changes, altering blood pressure and activating the hypothalamus. This leads to a parasympathetic response which balances your system. Do you remember where these type 3 and type 4 mechanoreceptors are in our body? Yes, they are in our jaw and in our digestive tract or our gut. (Schleip, R, 2003).

Many people today are diagnosed with IBS or irritable bowel syndrome. They are given a symptom-based diagnosis characterized by chronic abdominal pain, discomfort, bloating, and alteration of bowel habits. Type 3 and type 4 mechanoreceptors are in our gut, and they're responsible for our histamine levels which help us with inflammation of our gut. Michael Gershon in 1998 called the gut the second brain or the enteric nervous system (Gershon, Michael, 1998).

Louise Hay, author of *You Can Heal Your Life,* would ask those suffering from irritable bowel syndrome these questions: "What are you afraid to digest in life?" or "What are you holding onto" (Hay, L, 1982)?

People with irritable bowel syndrome are depressed all the time. They are often known to be constipated and have lower-than normal levels of serotonin. Serotonin is one of the most important neurotransmitters for the brain in your gut. It is crucial to the function of your digestive system. Your gut creates ninety five percent of the serotonin in your body. Serotonin changes the motility of your gut. It affects how sensitive your intestines are to sensations like pain and fullness. It helps us to feel awake, alert and good about ourselves (Case-Lo, C, 2012).

Appreciating serotonin's influences on the digestive system and the brain can help you understand the importance of having good posture. If you are constantly in poor posture, your diaphragmatic breathing is going to lesson, and this can have an effect on the motility of the gut. Remember, the diaphragm has a direct connection to the pelvic floor. Constricting energy to the pelvic floor may cause constipation. You might find depression increasing if you are unable to move your bowels.

I often think about my geriatric population and my special needs clients who spend long hours within their wheelchairs. Both populations sit in a forward flexed posture. We know that serotonin plays a huge role in the gut and with the breath, and that poor posture can possibly affect serotonin levels. We have to open up the diaphragm for these clients. It is important to get that working so that the digestive system works.

In Yoga, Tai Chi, and Pilates, the navel center is the energetic center. Now we know why it is for so many different reasons.

Let's talk about a study involving the connections among the hypothalamus, the pituitary gland, and the pineal gland. In May 2014, the *Journal of the American Physical Therapy Association* published an article titled "A Modern Neuroscience Approach to Chronic Spinal Pain: Combining Pain Neuroscience Education with Cognition Targeted Motor-Control Training." The article points out that there is brain atrophy – a decrease in the density of grey matter containing neural cell bodies – in chronic, low-back pain clients (Nijs, J., Meeus, M., Cagnie, B., Roussel, N. A., Dolphens, M., Van Oosterwijck, J., & Danneels, L, 2014).

The chronic pain clients I have treated are somewhat miserable, having given up hope that they will recover. Remember that the amygdala, the emotional center of the brain, can create imbalance in the hypothalamus, a nervous system and endocrine system gland. If you have chronic pain for a long time, I can guarantee that you won't always be so positive about life. In cases like this, the amygdala is constantly under attack, which creates shifts in the regulatory center of our brain, the hypothalamus. The fight or flight response is constantly turned on, making learning or retaining information a difficult task. Descending pain inhibition is malfunctioning as well. In fact, these clients show signs of central stabilization, an amplification of neural signaling within the central nervous system and have challenges in fine tuning movements during activities of daily living. Perhaps, if these clients can gain control of their pain, then the density of their gray matter would return back to normal.

In an article titled "A Modern Neuroscience Approach to Chronic Spinal Pain: Combining Pain Neuroscience Education with Cognition-Target Motor Control Training," the authors examined chronic spinal pain patients. It was found that these patients had brain atrophy, a decrease in the density of the gray matter of their brain. They discovered that by telling these patients to stop an exercise once it hurts – a system-contingent approach – didn't allow the patients to connect their mind to their bodies. The mind will always give up first and then the body will automatically stop. The mind requires direction ((Nijs, J., Meeus, M., Cagnie, B., Roussel, N. A., Dolphens, M., Van Oosterwijck, J., & Danneels, L, 2014).

A new approach now being used and discussed within this article is a time-contingent approach where patients perform the activity for five minutes regardless of the pain. In other words, work to control the mind so that it can be liberated. Using this modern neuroscience approach helped to decrease these patients' pain and also helped to reverse the brain atrophy within the gray matter of the brain.

This new approach is similar to yogic philosophy which believes that meditation minutes or a desired time is essential for mind and body effects.In my Kundalini yoga practice, the tools of breath work and meditation coupled with sound, eye focus, mudras, postures, and locks can change different avenues of the brain.

Yogic science says that there are particular lengths of time needed for desired affects during meditation (Bhagan Y, 2007). For example, thirty-one minutes of any type of meditation or breath work can affect your blood, your organs, and the rhythm of your cells. Every cell and every organ in our body has a certain frequency and vibration. The interesting news relating to healing is that doing sixty-two minutes of meditation/ breathing exercises daily can actually change the grey matter in your brain (Bhajan, Y, 2007). If clients with chronic pain used a yogic practice of meditation and breath-work, they could gain control of their pain, and of course, help their brain to heal. In fact, doing sixty-two minutes of a meditation/yogic set could help repair the gray matter in the brain.

The study also mentions creating motor-imagery – retraining the brain's circuitry responsible for successful completion of a recommended task – is a process that also needs to be included. That means addressing the client's cognitions and perceptions about the issue, discussing the anticipated consequences of the exercises, challenging the patients' cognitions in relation to the exercises, and then increasing the complexity of the exercises from static to dynamic/functional exercises.

In conclusion, the great thing about this research study is that clients can now learn to really connect with their pain and their body through their sensory system and formulate positive body language to successfully heal. They can't fail because through time they can reorganize and control their brain's response – particularly the mind – to the pain. This new approach to therapy is applicable to any client.

Herbert Benson is a well-known cardiologist and pioneer in the use of the breath in treatment. His work, written in *The Relaxation Response*, outlines his success with his clients using the breath in treatment. He found that thirty-four percent of people with chronic pain reduced their medication with meditation. Seventy-five percent of insomniacs were able to sleep normally. Long-term meditators experienced eighty percent less heart disease and fifty percent less cancer than non-meditators. He found that the breath also helps with hearing ability, blood pressure and vision, reactivation of melatonin and serotonin, reduced blood lactate, DHEA production, and improved oxygen levels during sleep. Herbert Benson's work is another prime example of the power of the breath (Khalsa, D.S., Stauth, C.).

Our thought patterns – how we think about ourselves – can be reflected within our physical body. Candace Pert, author of *Molecules of Emotions*, said that emotions aren't simply "I'm happy" or "I'm sad," but rather biochemical properties that interact with the brain to cause some type of response and produce feelings. She found that internal chemicals – neuropeptides and their receptors – are the biological components of our awareness, manifesting as beliefs, emotions, expectations and how we respond to the world (Pert, C, 1997).

The cells in our bodies are the basic structural and functional unit of the body. You can think of the cell as an engine that directs life. Receptors are like buttons on the control panel. These receptors are molecules made of protein that are able to recognize other molecules that hang around the cell membrane. On these receptors are ligands which act like fingers. They press the buttons to operate the cell. The ligands are neurotransmitters, steroids or peptides which are informational substances made up of strings of amino acids and neuropeptides or peptides active in neural tissue.

Our emotions are carried around the body by peptide ligands that bind to the receptors of each cell and can change the cell's chemical properties. The ligands can carry an electrical charge and can change the frequency and vibration of the cell. Certain cells may become glued to certain ligands – sad emotions or even angry emotions. So sometimes when you get sad and you wonder why you're sad, it may just be because the vibration of your cells is decreased. They are not vibrating as they should.

Today, antidepressants are widely used. When you take an anti-depressant it can definitely change the vibration of your cells. Your hope is that you may feel better. But then after about three months, you may notice that you are getting sad again and that the drug isn't working as well. You may be prescribed another anti-depressant, but this time you may be developing suicidal thoughts. This new anti-depressant has become addicted to your sad emotions, making you feel worse and glummer.

Instead of the anti-depressants, as mentioned earlier, there are neuropeptides in our respiratory system that can recharge us and help us vibrate better. Breathe and meditate and you can change your cellular vibration naturally and never have to be on drugs again. You can literally get a high on life by breathing in life.

There are many other studies that have shown that the use of yoga breathing is beneficial for helping with various disorders. Yoga breathing and yoga principles have proven successful with female fibromyalgia and breast cancer survivors. The results have shown success with pain management, better mood, relaxation, and acceptance for these clients (Wren AA, Wright, MA, Carson, JW, and Keefe, FJ, 2011).

Yoga and deep breathing have been used to address soldiers' post-traumatic stress. An estimated twenty percent of the two million Iraq and Afghanistan veterans suffer from post-traumatic stress. Twenty Wisconsin veterans participated in a study using meditation and deep breathing which helped them lower their heart rate and breathing rates. The long term effects included positive attitude and yoga follow-through. Now VA hospitals, such as those in Madison, Wisconsin are offering yoga and meditation classes (Jones, 2012).

A study from Roudebush Veteran's Administration Medical Center and from University of Indiana examined yoga programs with chronic stroke patients. Results showed less disability, improved balance, reduced fear of falling, and better quality of life with these clients. What's more, a study titled "Post Stroke Balance Also Improves with Yoga" assessed the impact of a yoga-based rehab intervention on balance, balance self-efficacy, fear of falling, and quality of life after stroke. Yoga sessions within this study occurred two times per week for eight weeks with a yoga therapist and included seated, standing, and floor postures and meditation and relaxation. Assessments used were the Berg Balance

Scale, Balance Confidence Scale, and the Stroke Quality of Life scale. The results showed that a group yoga-based rehab intervention for people with chronic stroke has potential in improving multiple post stroke variables and that group yoga may be possible in medical-based and community-based settings and may be cost effective. (Schmid, A, etc., 2012).

Yoga Helps with Asthma is another important study. This study included twenty individuals from twenty to sixty-five years old. One group practiced Hatha yoga for two and a half hours per week, holding poses for one minute and focusing on deep breathing. The other group was a non-yoga control group. The study lasted for a total of ten weeks. Heart rate variability and oxygen consumption were also assessed. Results were based on a questionnaire that measured frequency and severity of symptoms. Yoga enhanced awareness of breathing. The yoga group improved by forty-three percent (Gardner, 2009).

Another study was titled *The Effect of Yoga Training on Pulmonary Functions in Patients with Bronchial Asthma*. This study included yoga breathing exercises for group A with group B as the control group. One hundred twenty people were involved in the study. Pulmonary function tests were performed at baseline, at 4 weeks, and after eight weeks. Results of this study showed that yoga breathing exercises can be used adjunctively with standard pharmacological treatment, significantly improving pulmonary functions in patients with bronchial asthma (Sochi, C, Sing, S, Dandona, PK, 2009).

Lastly, research on the *Effect of Physiotherapy-Based Breathing Retraining on Asthma Control* was a six month controlled study involving forty adults with stable, mild to moderate asthma under the same specialist's care. Some adults, randomly, were trained in either twelve individual breathing retraining sessions or acted as the control group who received usual asthma care. The study used the Asthma Control Test, respiratory rate, spirometry, and scores from Nijmegen Hyperventilation Questionnaire, Medical Research Council scale, and Quality of Life Questionnaire. The results proved that breathing retraining results in improvements not only in asthma control but also in physiological factors across time (Grammatopoulou, EP, etc., 2011).

The mind is indeed instrumental in supporting the body's emotions and knowledge. Yet, remember, the body may be the controller of the mind for knowledge, and we should look at our bodies and not our minds first and foremost. Using proper breathing independently or in combination with yoga can enhance this mind-body connection and assist in self-healing.

Chapter 9: The Systems Model Approach

"The measure of greatness in a scientific idea is the extent to which it stimulates thought and opens up new lines of research."   Paul Dirac

There is a complex functional relationship between the muscles and the joints. You have now reached a point within this book where you can see that poor posture is linked to painful conditions in the extremities, balance disorders, poor endurance, decreased eyesight, behavioral changes, headaches, fear or anger, auditory impairments, and even temporal mandibular or jaw joint problems. Our connective tissue plays an integral role as a communication network that connects all the systems together. Therefore, today the body needs to be examined in its entirety – as an integrated, functional system. Descartes, the Father of Modern Philosophy and the formulator of Reductionism and Cartesian Thought, often said that reasoning comes from a general set of facts, broken down into to one specific, certain fact. In other words, with any complex idea or system, you had to break it down into its component parts and then put them together correctly.

In medicine today, the natural inclination seems to be to look at the single factors responsible for a problem in isolation – which has led to specialization. Physicians typically locate that secluded irregularity or single focus for medical management. It has become extremely difficult to reduce a client's pathology to single, isolated cause. As a result, Western doctors are often classified by their specialties, such as cardiology, gynecology, immunology, and so on. On the other hand, our current research and knowledge is holism: that the whole body, its organs and systems are linked (Khalsa, D.S. and Stauth, C, 2001).

Not only are our bodies connected, but we are all connected. We are all part of the same system. We will have to look at all the systems, including our mind and our cognition. Additionally, more than anything, we are going to have to really look at our connective tissue.

Mark Hyman's book called *Ultra Prevention* is an absolutely eye opening text with some fabulous information about nutrition and health. He cites a study reported by the American Medical Association Journal about on the average time doctors spend with their clients.

Any guesses? The average time spent is about twenty three seconds before either the doctor has selected a diagnosis from his/her medical book or before an interruption takes place. The doctor may already think he or she knows what the problem is before actually looking at the client's actual situation. The doctor already has a recipe and the doctor knows exactly what it is. I have one question. Does this allow enough time for the body to be evaluated in its entirety?

Here are some examples of how I, as a physical therapist, learned to see outside the box. A male physical therapist attended one of my yoga courses and said to me that previously he did not believe in yoga, but just recently yoga had changed his life. He reported that he had a history of heart, thyroid, and digestive issues and was constantly on medications. He was also depressed all the time. He attended a yoga class and the instructor worked on nasal breathing. He claimed that after the yoga class, he was able to breathe better and felt better within his body.

He searched for an ENT doctor, an ear, nose, and throat specialist. When he went to the ENT doctor, he was told he had a deviated septum. He proceeded to have surgery to correct his deviated septum, and it cured all of his medical issues. He was off all his medications and discovered the practice of yoga as his new therapy.

Remember, the nasal septum is responsible for the secretion and balancing of our cerebrospinal fluid. Each side of the nose is innervated by five different cranial nerves, each responsible for dehumidifying the air and helping with our energy levels. It would be well worth any therapist's time to check out all the latest research about how breathing techniques can help deviated septum clients.

My mother, on the other hand is a perfect example of the negative impact of not having her entire body evaluated. After my mom underwent two total knee surgeries and was in a post-rehabilitation facility in Illinois, she was still suffering with pain. I received a phone call from her and immediately flew to Illinois to give her support. Although she was receiving ongoing physical therapy at a very reputable orthopedic outpatient facility, my mother expressed to me that she felt like she was behind in her healing process.

Mother started developing foot problems aside from her knee issues and asked me if the knee and foot were connected. I, of course, said "Yes." I said to her that after any knee surgery the body changes. Your walk changes because the new knee alignment will now impact the foot placement. The foot may hit the ground differently causing compensation patterns all over the body. The feet always should be evaluated after a total knee replacement surgery.

My mother was not convinced. How many of you have parents who ask you questions and, although you may be an expert in your field, they never pay attention to you, but they will listen to someone else?

So I proceeded to shut my mouth and went with my mother to her physical training sessions. I'll never forget one of her sessions. My mother asked the physical therapist the same question she asked me earlier that morning. The PT said to her that the knee is not connected to her foot. He then proceeded to ignore my mother's questions and her hurt feelings and spent 15 minutes performing joint mobilizations techniques on her knee. Then he gave her a quick knee massage.

I asked my mom, "Has this physical therapist ever looked at your gait?"

She said, "No, no, no."

Soon after the therapist left, an assistant came over and took my mother to the exercise room to do her exercise program. I watched my mother perform her program with little connection to her body, no breathing, and just doing the exercises to do them. The assistant wasn't paying much attention to my mother. Her job was simply reading off the exercise program and checking off the exercises my mom completed. After ten minutes of watching this painful experience, I couldn't take it anymore. The assistant clearly was not giving my mother feedback and my mother looked like she was suffering from poor posture.

So I said to this nice girl, "Are you going to give my mom cues? Are you going to tell her about the breath?"

She replied, "Well, I just started here like last week. They haven't trained me yet."

I'm thinking "Oh, my Goodness!" I mean, this is a really reputable place, but she shouldn't be working without proper training.I said to her, "Can I help you with my mother, and I will teach you how to work with her so she has good posture and is using her own body senses and her breath."

How did this session end up for my mother? The assistant said to me, "Thank you so much. I learned more from you in the last thirty minutes than I've learned from the facility that actually hired me."

I am not saying that a lot of facilities are like this because that's not the case, but the question is, are clients getting quality care? Are we just focused on one body segment, or are we in such a hurry to get these clients in and out that we neglect seeing the entire picture?

My mother soon started letting me help her rehabilitate her body. I chose a systems model approach to her treatment. Her ankle problem and her knee pain all diminished. She became aware of her body and what her body actually needed. The greatest gift is that her body gave her all the internal answers that she needed, lessening her reliance on others for help.

The Influence of Body-based Psychology

Somatic Psychology, also known as Body-based Psychology – a new field of study – is based on the premise that the body cannot lie and that we can trust in the innate wisdom of the body. All psychological processes occur within the body and psychological patterns have physical components. A therapist involved in this field observes where there is movement or fixation in a body part and then uses the information to guide the clients' processes by looking at body sensations, emotions, and thoughts and teaching the client to gain awareness within their body.

Wilhelm Reich, the father of Somatic Psychology in the 1930's, was influenced by the work of Freud. He based his theories on muscular armor and character structure. He looked at energy and how it flows through the body, similar to the Eastern medical practices of Yoga, acupuncture and acupressure. Energy, he comments, flows smoothly with healthy individuals but can be blocked in neurotic and psychotic clients (Foster, MA.). His goal was to be able to connect all the processes – mental, emotional, and psychological.

His breakthrough in this field came when he was working with a client who was able to release suppressed rage. So how did Wilhelm Reich do this? He identified that the client had muscular armoring or chronic muscular tension around his jaw area. Wilhelm Reich placed his hands on the client's jaw and massaged it more and more deeply. Then he asked the client to breathe and to focus on his jaw area. As he moved deeper, the client released all of his anger. The client's pain, physical and mental, dissipated. He was holding all this anger and his past within his jaw. Perhaps, he had been too afraid all these years to use his voice to express his anger, and it was just held in this jaw area. The deeper Wilhelm Reich went with his hands, the deeper he was able to touch the client's hidden emotions.

It seems that when we give attention to a problem, we are given an opportunity to change or grow. Remember my client Dee? Because of her knee pain, she searched for ways to alleviate it. Dee, if you recall, liked to lean and shift her weight toward the right side. Because of her lack of motion in her right ankle joint, the left side of her body, particularly her left knee, was a big point of stress, especially during walking. Dee saw nothing wrong with her walking and never noticed how much she leaned to the right.

Her awakening came when I asked her to walk and lean to the right. Since she was already imbalanced, this task made her extremely unstable, causing her to almost fall to the right. Because of this, she recognized her body's movement pattern and was willing to correct it.

Going deeper into a problem, whether it is to address a mobility skill created by neglect or just habit, as in Dee's case, or tightening a muscle that is already tight by breathing into that muscle in order to feel and recognize where the pain is coming from are ways of opening and awakening up the body so change can occur.

Body-based Psychology, therefore, monitors the relationships among body sensations and emotions or psychological issues. The goals are to assist the client in letting go of holding patterns within their body and to release muscular armor, restoring normal flow or movement within the body. This may entail deep tissue massage, deep breathing exercises, and moving a client toward their resistive pattern.

Two examples of bands of armor that occur within the body are located in the ocular or eye region and the abdominal region. The ocular segment is around the eyes and tells us that a client may have issues about not wanting to see something. Rolling the eyes and encouraging movement of the eyes can help melt away ocular armor. The abdominal segment conveys that the client may have fears about life or, in fact, is afraid to digest life. They may have constipation issues, refusing to release old ideas. Diaphragmatic breathing along with an abdominal massage may dissipate this type of armoring (Foster, M.A).

Bonnie Bainbridge Cohen, developer of Body/Mind Centering, expresses that we need to have a personal relationship with our body, especially the inside of our body. She worked with dance teachers to help them understand the importance of learning about the anatomy of the body and the connective tissue planes within the body. By convincing these teachers that this was not detrimental but rather beneficial to the dancers, she changed their perspectives. They soon realized that understanding the body in its entirety created more flow within the dancers' movement and greater body awareness.

In fact, Bonnie Bainbridge Cohen had her own personal experience with this viewpoint. When she was giving birth, her baby was breech. Apparently her doctors were concerned and were going to perform a C-section. Feeling connected with her baby and her body, she got on her hands and knees and felt the movement pattern of her baby. She gave birth to her baby in this position, and it was not born breech.

My goal, and probably yours, is to get to a level where we have such a strong relationship and connection to the "I" within us so that all the answers we need for healing can be internally felt and sensed.

You have come to a point in this chapter where I hope you realize that most models of care are now converting to a systems-based, integrative model. A systems model allows us to look deeper into the cause of a problem without immediately making an assumption or judgment. This involves not only using our senses – hearing, vision, smell, taste, and touch – but also peering into the mechanisms of the mind – behaviors, cognition, emotions, memory, and stress. Of course, the motor and skeletal systems – the bones, connective tissue, fascia, and muscles – also need to be addressed.

Mapping the Body Connections

In a manner similar to the way that cell phones have made communication easier and faster in the world today, understanding of our fascial system has expanded our knowledge and communication within our body to a deeper level. We owe thanks to Tom Meyers, author of *Anatomy Trains,* who has brilliantly mapped out fascial planes and given the world an understanding of how the body is connected. His article, *Early Dissective Evidence* published in 2006, outlines these fascial lines. His work has given me a new perspective on how to treat problems within the body by tracing the entire pathway of the injury site, from the head all the way to the bottom of the feet.

I'm most familiar with Tom Meyer's Superficial Back Line. The Superficial Back Line can be compared to the Life Nerve in my Kundalini yoga practice. This line is very significant because it is responsible for the development of our spine into extension so we can walk and keep our heads upright. It also helps with our overall mobility, balance, and coordination. This line attaches from the plantar fasciitis at the bottom of the foot; then to the ankle, the calf, the soleus and gastrocnemius, the hamstrings and the back muscles, all the way to the top of the head and to the scalp fascia. The Life Nerve continues its journey and ends at the third-eye point located between the brows. Becoming aware of this line and its connections to each body part can help in the treatment of hamstring problems, plantar fasciitis, back pain, and visual issues.

For example, when treating a client with headaches, you should think about examining the bottom of the foot, the hamstrings, the lower back, and the third eye point.

You should be looking for muscle or fascial tightness and whether the client is breathing correctly. If the diaphragm is not activated, then the lower back musculature will not get innervated, and therefore, all the muscles and fascia attached to the back can become affected. This example should prove to you that looking at the body involves stepping out of the box and not just examining one particular body part because, as you can see, everything is connected.

To counterbalance the Superficial Back Line is the Superficial Front Line which connects the entire anterior surface of the body. This line is responsible for creating flexion of the trunk and hips, extension of the knees, and dorsiflexion or backward bending of the foot which is similar to a baby's posture within the womb. This line stems from the mastoid process of the jaw to the sternocleidomastoid muscle of the neck to the rectus abdominis (abdominal muscles); then to the anterior/inferior iliac spine (the bony eminences on the anterior borders of the hip bones) to the rectus femoris (quadriceps muscles), the knee cap or patella, and ends at the dorsal phalanges of the feet (top of the feet).

When you are thinking outside the box, you would notice if a client who has TMJ issues has tight musculature or fascia anywhere along this line and thus, the cause of the problem may not be TMJ, but perhaps tight abdominal muscles. Treat the abdominal area and the TMJ issue may dissipate.

When I asked you early on to squeeze the fourth and fifth digits, recall what happened to your posture? The answer was that you were able to bring your shoulders back so your posture became more upright. The fourth and fifth digits are part of Tom Meyer's Arm Line. This is the deep arm line he talks about, and he reveals that this line runs from the fourth and fifth digits all the way up the arm, along the triceps to the scapular area where the rhomboids, the levator scapulae, and the serratus anterior muscles are located. These scapular muscles are responsible for bringing the shoulders back and helping with upright posture. Can you see that a client with scapular pain or tightness would benefit from work along the triceps area and hand area?

Tom Meyers also talks about the Lateral Line, the line that assists movement between the Superficial Front Line and Superficial Back Line and counterbalances them. The muscles and bones included are the mastoid process or the jaw, the ribs, the gluteus maximus and medius muscles (buttock muscles), the iliotibial tract (the thick band on the side of the leg that attaches from the pelvis to the shin bone) , the fibular head (the bony eminence on outside of the lower leg), the peroneal muscles(muscles on lateral compartment of shin, responsible for the turning out of your foot) and the 1 and 5 metatarsal bones (bones of the feet).

Here are some examples of how to use the Lateral Line in diagnosis. If you have a client with jaw issues, are you treating their IT band? Are you looking at their glutes? Are you looking at the peroneal muscles along their leg to counterbalance what's going on in the jaw? If a client came in with a dropped foot or a collapsed arch, are you addressing tightness at the buttock muscles, jaw, and rib cage.

Finally, the most important line is the Deep Front Line, the Core. I have spoken about this line throughout this book. This line encompasses the organs, muscles, bones, and fascia. It connects the jaw muscles, the diaphragm, the lumbar vertebral bodies (bones of the lower back), the psoas (rope like muscle deep in the belly, responsible mainly for hip flexion), iliacus (a triangular muscle that fills the iliac fossa on the interior of the hip bone), the lessor trochanter of the femur (part of hip bone) , the pelvic floor, the adductor magnus (muscles of the inner thigh), the medial femoral epicondyle (part of the medial side of the knee joint, a bony protrusion), the posterior tibia/fibula (the back of the lower leg), the plantar tarsal bones (bones on bottom of feet), and the plantar surface of the toes (bottom of toes). This is the most important line because it helps lift the inner arch, balances the neck and head, helps with breathing, stabilizes each segment of the leg, counterbalances lift to the pull of both the Superficial Front Line and Superficial Back Line, and helps with the rhythm of walking. So if a client's has problems with arch support, too much medial or lateral rotation of the knees, pelvic floor issues, swallowing issues, jaw issues, facial asymmetry and umbilicus asymmetry, tight psoas muscles, and even tight hamstrings, this is the fascial line where work needs to occur.

In therapeutic practice, try holding any of the following points along this deep core line (the jaw, the inside of the knee, the psoas, and the inside of the bottom of the foot) for five minutes. The client can then be instructed to perform conscious breathing through these points and asked to repeat positive affirmations for healing. The results can be amazing. The diaphragm becomes activated, reopening any blocks along this fascial line. The client then releases muscular and emotional tension and armoring.

The Acupressure Connection

Since we are speaking of pressing points within the body, acupressure is an ancient healing art using the fingers to press key healing points within the body. Acupuncture uses needles along these points or channels of energy called meridians, while acupressure uses gentle to firm finger pressure. There is even a new technique practiced by physical therapists called dry needling that uses needles for therapy of muscle pain or pain related to myofascial pain syndrome. Regardless of the slight differences between these three modalities, they all do not treat any particular pathological symptom, but really help normalize physiological homeostasis and promote self-healing. They all work to help treat the body as a whole (MA, Y and M, and Cho, ZH, 2005).

In 1990 Michael Gach wrote a great book called *Acupressure's Potent Points*. It is a wonderful way to learn how to use acupressure on yourself and others to relieve stress-related problems and other ailments that have created anxiety and tension within the body. Of course it is not intended as a substitute for the medical advice of a physician. I personally have used this book to advance my understanding in acupressure.

In his book, Gach has included 43 different chapters on common health issues. For example, if you wake up one morning and you say, "I have a headache," there is a chapter on headaches which shows you important potent points or acupressure points for relieving headaches and migraines. He includes pictures as a visual aid as well as a description of the potent point's benefits. He also recommends that conscious breathing should be used in connection with each potent point held. The book also explains that finger pressure should be used in a slow rhythmic manner. Every point should be held for two to three minutes, eventually working up to ten minutes. Avoid the abdominal area if the client has a life threatening disease, like intestinal cancer; also avoid this area if pregnant.

I find interesting correlations between my yogic practice and this Eastern modality, acupressure. Michael Gach speaks about two main things that he does as part of his daily routine. One of these rituals is rubbing both of his ears. He explains that there are over 150 meridians, energy centers or pathways, located on the ear. The whole body is also reflected in the ear according to Chinese medicine. If you look at the ear, it represents an upside down fetus with the head of the fetus toward the ear lobe and the body toward the top of the ear. By massaging the ear and holding points along the ear, you are actually massaging the entire body.

The second ritual that he does is an exercise or yogic posture called spinal flexion, which you will be able to experience in a little bit. Spinal flexion will open all the meridians along the back region.

Let's learn a couple of these points so that we can begin to use these points as tools to help us heal. You will see that these points all link together to the fascial pathways and even to the yogic mudras and energy centers.

If you remember, the most important point in the body related to the core and from where movement should originate is right below the navel point. With acupressure, this point is called the Sea of Energy or CV 6, one of the most energetic points in our body. Locate it two finger widths directly below the belly button. Hold this point and consciously breathe into it. It will help relieve lower back weakness, tone weak abdominal muscles, and prevent a variety of lower-back problems. It will also lessen pain in the abdominal muscles and help with constipation, colitis, and gas.

If a client or someone you know suffers from acid reflux or has lower back problems, merely have them lie on their back, and either have them place their fingers on this area and consciously breathe or use a hockey puck or object and place it on this area and have them breathe. Using objects, like a hockey puck, are great visual aids and assist in providing tactile cuing to the body. In fact, you can place a hockey puck on the sea of energy area, on the chest area, and on the clavicular or collarbone area. I observe my clients breathing. When my clients have a hard time filling up the abdominal area, the chest area, and the clavicular area when they inhale, these objects assist them to activate these areas. Once these areas are activated, the hockey puck will rise up and the clients will get immediate body feedback. This will be discussed further in the next chapter.

CV 6 Point or Sea of Energy

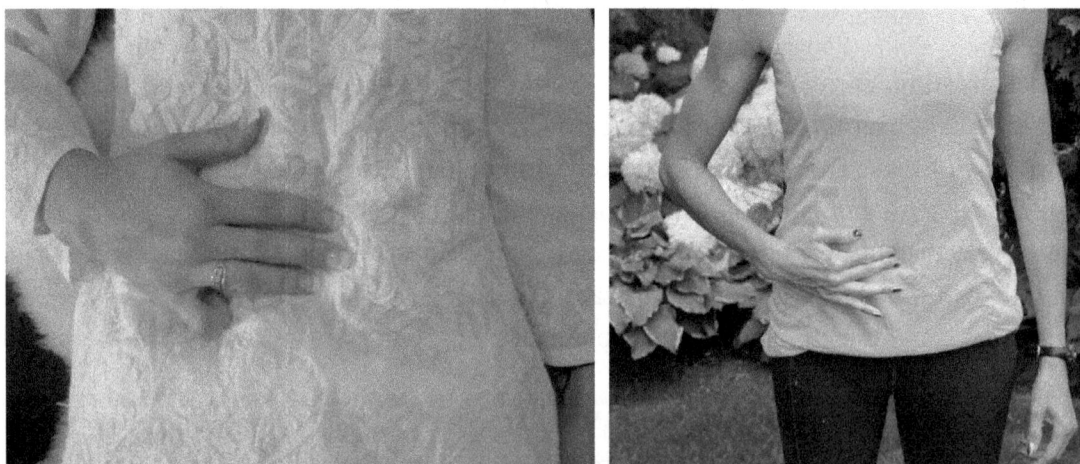

B54 or Commanding Middle is another great potent point. It is located in the center of the back of the knee crease (Gach, M.R., 1990). Lie on the floor for a moment and place your fingers on this location. You will have to bring your knees up to your chest, and use gentle, firm pressure on this point.

As an aside, I'm a Reiki practitioner and sometimes I don't even put my hands directly on a client's body. Did you know that you can work on someone's body even ten feet away? The heat from my hands can guide me to areas of the body where there is resistance or tension. These are often the areas that need attention.

Keep in mind that if you push too hard on the body, the body will resist and prevent you from entering it. This is probably a self-protective mechanism. At least, this is what I have experienced in my practice. Work with each individual's system. Listen to each bodily system, and the system will guide you to where it needs relief and how much pressure to employ on it.

The Commanding Middle or B 54 will relieves back pain, sciatica, knee pain, back stiffness, and arthritis in the knees, back, and the hips. When I work with clients with spinal issues, I have them lie on the ground, bring their knees to their chest, and place their fingers on the Commanding Middle point. Of course they will also be doing deep abdominal breathing. They can even gently do back rolls while they are in this same position, holding this point, and slowly rocking forward and backwards, giving the back a gentle massage.

B 54 or Commanding Middle

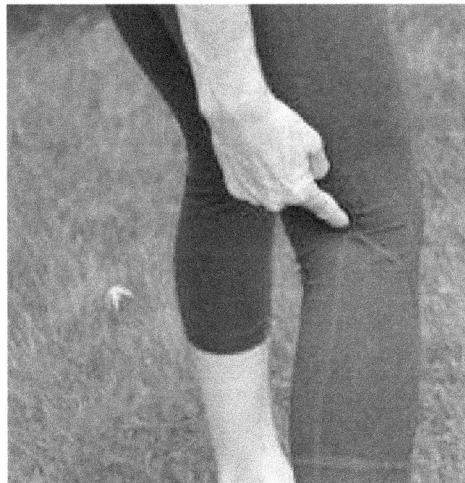

Back rolls: Correct way and incorrect way – Activating B 54

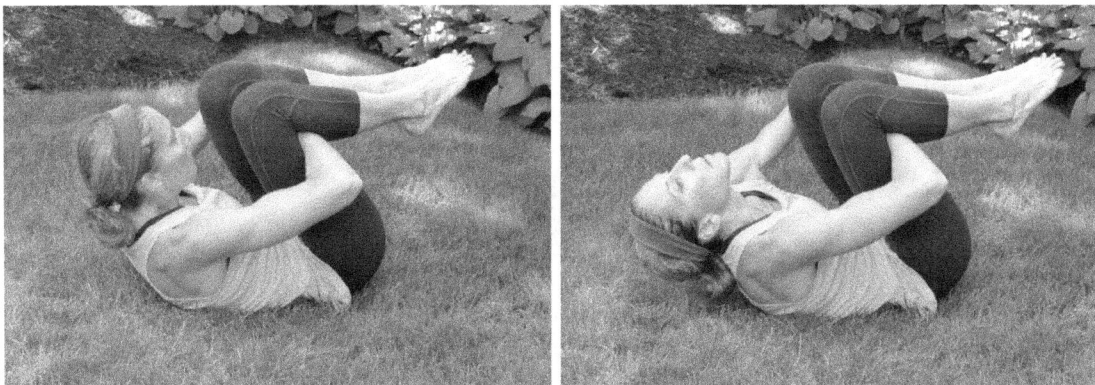

The third eye point or GV 24.5 is another point used in acupressure. The yogis use this point for eye focus to help open the pituitary gland and to help with intuition. According to fascial lines and yogic meridians, the life nerve originates at the bottom of the feet and attaches to the third eye point. The significance of the third eye point, located between the eyebrows, is that it assists the endocrine system, especially the pituitary gland. It also aids in easing hay fever, headaches, and eye strain. If you are undergoing eye strain or eye issues, you can actually hold this point and do some deep breathing to let go of this pain.

In yogic practice, the baby pose emphasizes that the third eye point touches the ground, not the forehead as some have thought. This opens the pituitary gland and balances the hypothalamus, the regulating center of the brain. Baby pose received its name because it was intended to stop temper tantrums by self-containing the body and bringing the focus back to the breath in order to slow down the fight or flight response.

Third eye point or GV 24.5

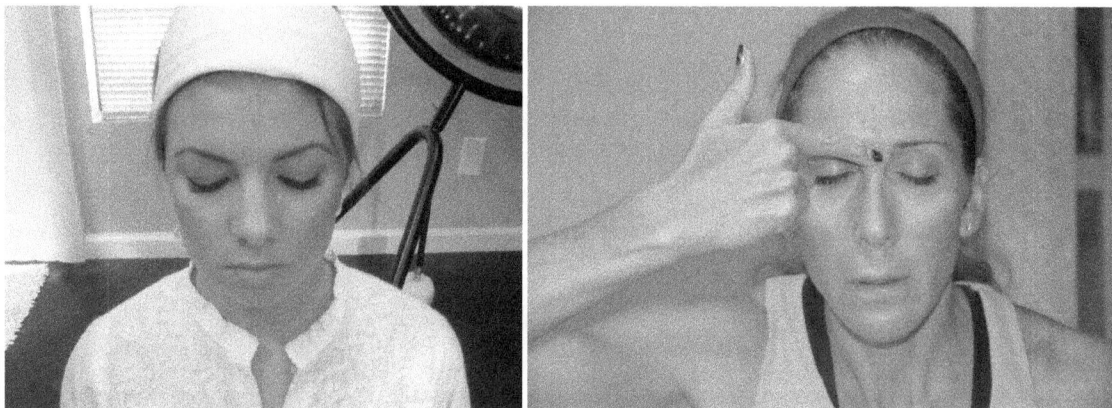

Baby Pose

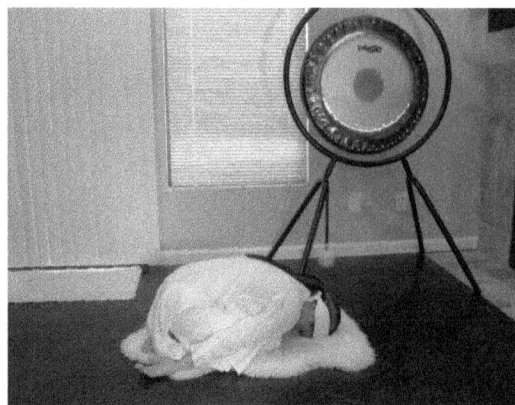

What is the most common hand position used for prayer? It is called the prayer pose. I mentioned prayer pose earlier in this book. With prayer pose, you use both your right and left hand which balances masculine and feminine energy or negative and positive energy. Place your hands at the center of the breastbone, three finger widths from the base of the bone. Michael Gach calls this point the Sea of Tranquility or CV 17. By pushing on this point and breathing, you're going to actually help relieve nervousness, anxiety, chest tension, anguish, depression, hysteria, and other emotional imbalances.

I have my clients who see me for the first time place their hands in prayer pose, close their eyes, and perform some deep breathing. This is very balancing and creates stillness within the body, erasing fears and tension. It creates neutrality between both parties, allowing the client to feel safe in this new environment and connected to his or her self. Being within this sacred space provides opportunities for transformation.

CV 17 or Sea of Tranquility

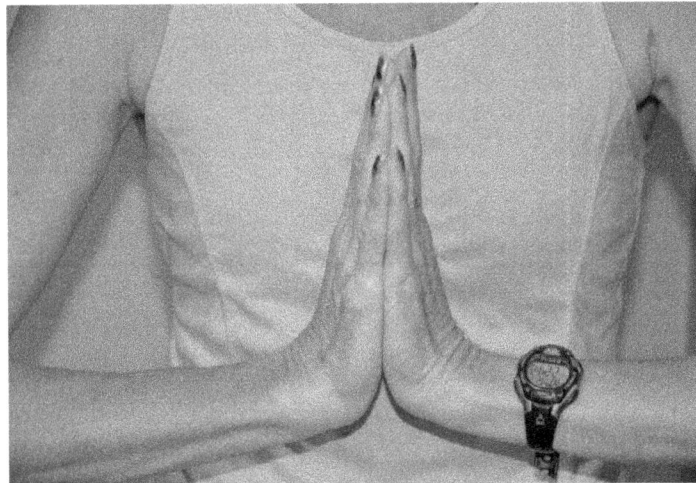

Michael Gach also describes the use of the K 27 point or Elegant Mansion. This point is located in the hollow where the collarbone and the sternum meet, right underneath the collarbone. The significance of this point is that it relieves chest congestion, breathing difficulties, asthma, coughing, and anxiety. Think about using this point to help yourself if you are experiencing anxiety or nervousness. I use this point all the time on my clients. I have some clients who are on respiratory systems for breathing and some who have severe scoliosis so that they really can't use their arms. Some of my clients have both of these ailments. If these clients have difficulty with diaphragmatic breathing, I try to help them. I hold the Elegant Mansion point and then wait for a few minutes. I see the diaphragm automatically begin moving.

I work with a client with scoliosis who has a 70 degree curve where you can actually see the hip bone and rib cage touching. The side where this is occurring usually is where the diaphragm is slightly compressed. I initially position this client in sideline (on their side) opposite the side that is compressed. I then use the Elegant Mansion point and hold it there. The diaphragm on the side that is compressed will become activated and soon the breath becomes equalized on both sides.

K 27 or Elegant Mansion

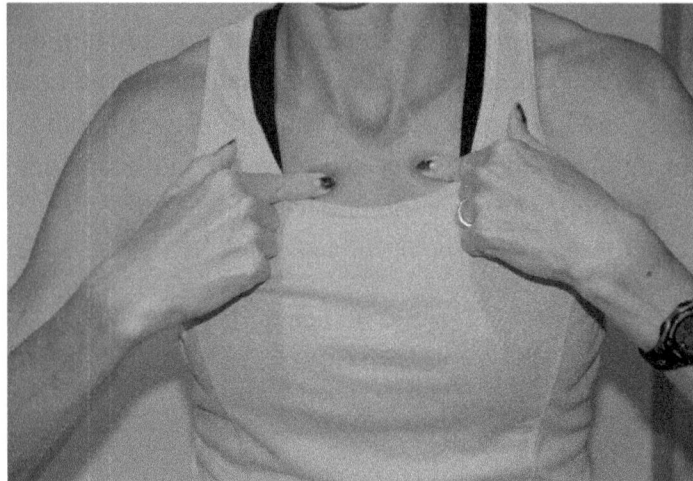

Lastly, GB 20 or Gate of Consciousness Point is located below the base of the skull, in the hollows which are two to three inches apart, depending on the size of the head. This point diminishes jaw pain, headaches, stiff necks, and neck pain. It is amazing how fast I can relieve a headache using my own body just by leaning up against the back of a chair, placing the base of my skull against these points, and executing conscious breathing.

GB 20 or Gates of Consciousness

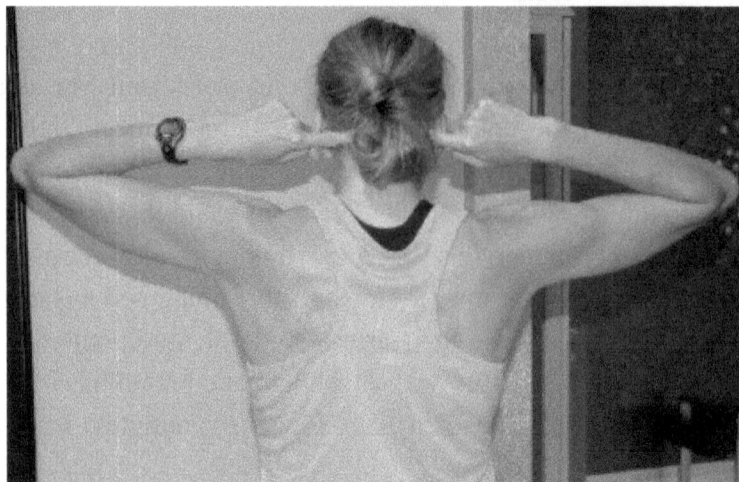

Increased Popularity of Integrative Medicine

Currently, more health care practitioners seem interested in using integrative medicine within their practice. Do you ever watch the Dr. Oz show? It is a great show with some excellent ideas about health and wellness.

Dr. Soram Khalsa was featured on this show. He is an integrative medical doctor who really aims to get his patients well. He explains that one's state of health is on a spectrum, from disease to wellness. Dr. Khalsa encourages more doctors to become more multidisciplinary and be more open in their ideas from what they are taught by thinking outside the box. In his own practice, he applies all kinds of modalities, including acupuncture, herbal medicine, and kinesiology testing. He encourages doctors and other health practitioners to use more integrative medicine within their practice and to research the Institute of Functional Medicine.

It is very refreshing to see the doorway to integrative medicine opening. There is a collective consciousness shift occurring within humanity. More people are becoming awake to their own personal spiritual practice and are seeking more integrated medicine treatments for self-healing.

One particular modality of healing, Reiki, a form of palm healing or hands-on healing, is now being used in some hospital systems. In Arizona, some of our hospitals have Reiki practitioners who visit clients before and after surgery or who assist in any process of healing. A study titled "Reiki Treatment Helps Heart Attack Patients" used a twenty minute Reiki treatment within three days after a client suffered a heart attack. The result showed improved mood and heart rate variability compared with control groups who were just resting or listening to music (Burg, M., Miles, P., Lee, F. and Lampert, R., 2010).

I'd like to share my own personal story about how Reiki has helped me. Two years ago, I suffered from a bout of kidney stones. For those of you who have never experienced kidney stones, it is a most horrific pain. The pain, I can honestly say, was definitely worse than giving birth naturally to my son. I woke up one morning and was literally in a flexed position on the floor in intense pain. My husband offered to take me to the hospital. In previous times when I had kidney stones, I was taken to the hospital where I would have to wait for six hours while being on morphine, and then told to go home and try to pass the stones on my own.

I refused the hospital but insisted that he take me to my Reiki teacher. She performed a two hour Reiki session on me. Within those two hours, she was able to break up my kidney stones using her hands and alleviate all my pain. Reiki proved to be an overall better choice in my case since I knew what to expect and had experienced kidney stones in the past.

Integrating Kundalini Yoga with Physical Therapy

Being a Kundalini Yoga teacher, I'd like to share with you how this yogic model integrates so nicely with other modalities. If you haven't seen or heard about this form of yoga, you will learn about it now. In my field of physical therapy, yogic and breathing modalities are being used to alleviate pain and help with stress and tension. There is more information about this in the research section of the book. (See chapters 8 and 10).

Kundalini Yoga is real Eastern yoga, brought to the United States by Yogi Bhajan. I do regret how yoga in the Western world has become so focused on the physical body that there is little emphasize on the breath. Unfortunately as Westerners, we get caught up in how we look.

I had been to numerous yoga classes prior to learning about Kundalini Yoga, and I will tell you that in other yoga classes, I was more concerned whether I was doing the posture correctly and if I did it better than the person next to me than actually going within and connecting all parts of myself. My ego and my judgment always got the best of me. I would stare at myself in a mirror while in a posture, and I didn't breathe because I was afraid I'd lose my balance. In fact, currently, I have treated clients with neck and back issues arising from hyper-extending themselves in a yoga class.

Kundalini yoga involves listening to your body, going within and experiencing a new journey of self. The journey encompasses experiencing a lot of emotions but there is always a transformation of some sort and blessings at the end.

Yoga actually means awareness. It really means the union of the individual's consciousness to the infinite. We are all our own teachers. We have our own tools for healing. We just need to use them to reflect on making our own bodily changes.

Every cell and organ in our body has its own cycle and pulse that exists in resonant harmony and sympathy to the cycles of the Earth and planets, helping us connect to our divine self. Our cells resonate both positively and negatively. When we lose our connection to the rhythms and cycles of nature and to the interconnection to things within the universe, this disharmony manifests as imbalances and disease within the body (Carey, D, 2002). Through the practice of yoga, meditation, sounds, eye focus, locks, postures, breath and mudras, we can access the core energetic systems within the body. In the human body, vitality refers to the energy moving from the sacrum and coccyx through the spine and to the back of the head or brain.

When you leave a Kundalini Yoga class, you should never feel real soreness or pain. Instead, you should feel like you are high on life and calm within your body. The reason for this is because if you are doing yoga correctly and if you are doing the breath work correctly, you can actually change your brain-wave patterns.

During proper brainwave functioning, the brain undergoes transitions from wakefulness to sleep. Our brain cycles during every single moment of time through different wave patterns. If you were listening to a teacher and obtaining information, your beta waves would be activated at their highest frequency. That is considered active, waking consciousness with your eyes open.

Our ultimate goal in Kundalini Yoga is to reach the alpha brain-wave state. The alpha brain-wave state is associated with states of relaxation where your eyes are closed as well as daydreaming with your eyes open and where you can still maintain awareness. This alpha brain-wave state helps sift out extraneous sensory inputs in the brain. Without proper filtering, the ability to execute many cognitive tasks can be challenging.

One of the questions I often get after teaching a yoga class is why do I feel high or kind of out of it? I explain that your brain wave state has changed to an alpha frequency and you may feel like you are in a state of total shunia – neutrality or zero point – a place of stillness and relaxation. I encourage that my students drink water or eat something prior to leaving my class. Being in this state can make you feel emotional or loopy in a positive way. It is like you just gave your entire body a massage, removing any toxins, tensions or stresses, both emotional and physical.

An interesting study in 2001 explored the physiological correlates of a highly practiced Kundalini Yoga meditator. It examined thoracic and abdominal breathing patterns, heart rate, skin conductance level and blood volume during pre-baseline, mediation, and post baseline periods. The results were astounding. A shift in breathing patterns may have contributed to the development of alpha EEG during meditation and an increase in theta EEG activity immediately following the meditation. Data showed a decrease in respiration from 11 breaths per min pre and 13 breaths per min post to a mean of 5 breaths per min during meditation (Arambula, P., Kawakami, M. and Gibray, K.H.,2001).

The yoga sutras compiled by Patanjali around 400 A.D. are the goals, philosophy, and structure of yoga and meditation discipline. These eight limbs of the yoga sutras work together in a coordinated way, similar to my physical therapy practice. Let's see how?

If a client comes to see me, they may say "I don't want to have pain anymore. I don't want to feel this crummy anymore. I just can't take it." This is the first limb, Yamas- the Don'ts. Usually, a client will either want to get rid of pain or some kind of physical ailment.

Then the client will say, "I do want to lose weight. And I do want to run that race that I was set to do. And I do want to love myself a little bit better." This is the second limb, the Niyama- the Do's. At this stage, the mind becomes clear. There are goals being made and the mind has a road map to follow.

Next, as a therapist, you're going to say, "Okay, so I understand your problem and I've figured out the cause. Now I'm going to give you some exercises that I want you to take home." So we call that the third limb, the Asanas. Asanas are physical postures or exercises. You may assign an exercise to a client to be done as a home program. But before you give the exercise, you need to incorporate the breath with the exercise. The fourth limb is the breath or Pranayam. You may say to the client, you're going to incorporate the breath with the exercise for five minutes which is a time-contingent approach.

The client may become distracted. The fifth state is called Pratayahar, synchronization of senses and thoughts. This limb is difficult for most clients. Let me share an example of this limb.

I was in a birthing class prior to giving birth to my son. The birthing instructor said, "Today you're going to learn about nutrition. You're going to learn about Pratayahar. You're going to learn about nutrition and its importance in staying healthy and eating right during pregnancy." She continued, "I'm giving each of you an orange. I want you to spend 20 minutes with your orange."

I raised my hand and said, "I don't have five minutes to eat lunch, let alone spend 20 minutes with an orange."

She said, "You need to experience this." Of course, all the students are looking at each other, confused. She closes the door, dims the light, and she says, "Okay, goodbye."

I don't know if any of my readers have spent 20 minutes with an orange before, but it was a great meditation for me. It was all very sensory related – listening, seeing, smelling and touching. I learned a lot about myself – eating healthy, and staying connected with a task without being interrupted. Did you know that even when people go to yoga classes, they are often distracted by a certain sound within or outside of the room or maybe a funny scent? Mastery of this fifth limb will eliminate any outside distractions because your senses and thoughts will be in sync so you are able to concentrate on the activity or task at hand.

The sixth limb, Dharana, is a single-point concentration that occurs when you are in a state of meditation. The breath is circulating throughout your body and you are focused. In physical therapy, when a client is doing his/her exercise program, the client will have reached a state of concentration or focus to where his/her breathing will become automatic and no outside distractions will occur.

You then move into Dhyana, the seventh limb, which is deep meditation. Here for example, the above client connects at a deeper level with the_exercise to the point where he/she becomes aware of the breath, and the body naturally settles into the exercise with ease.

Finally you reach Samadi, the eighth limb, which is oneness or awakening. At this point, your brain wave changes to an alpha frequency. Now that same client will be doing the exercise as if the body and mind are doing the exercise on their own, unconsciously. His/her breathing will slow down and the brain waves will reach that alpha brain wave state. Everything within the body flows and is without tension. Your goal as a therapist is to get the client to move into these last three stages – the stages of self-discovery and letting go.

The Origin of the Caduceus

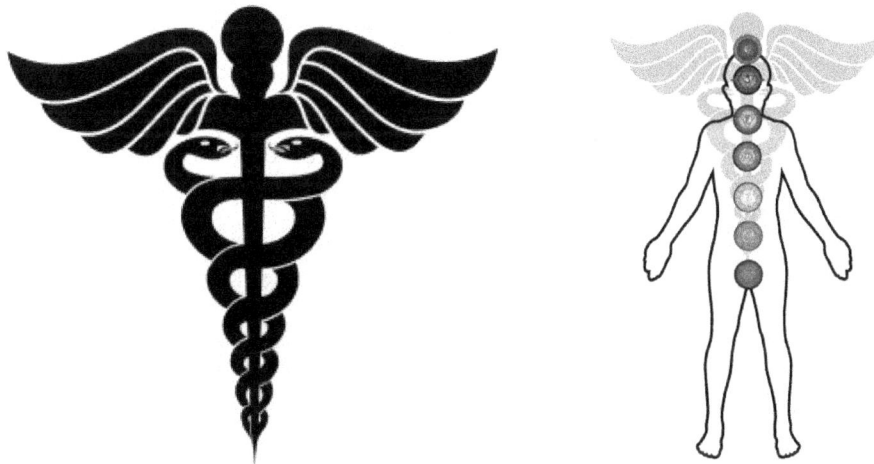

Understanding the Caduceus

Have you ever really analyzed the medical symbol of the caduceus and what it represents? Have you ever wondered who might have designed this symbol of two snakes, twining together on a pole, with wings at the top?

One possible explanation for the origin of this symbol dates back to the biblical story of Moses: "Then the Lord told Moses to make a metal snake and put it on a pole, so that anyone who was bitten [by a snake] could look at it and be healed. So Moses made a bronze snake and put it on a pole. Anyone who had been bitten would look at the bronze snake and be healed." (Numbers 21:8-9, Good News Version).

In Greek mythology, Hermes, the Olympian god, was a messenger between the gods and humans. He was also the supporter of travelers, which makes his link to medicine understandable because in the past doctors would have to travel long distances on foot to visit their patients (Melina, R, 2011). Another idea is that this image was borrowed from the yogis many, many thousands of years ago. Today, this image is seen all over the world, representing modern medicine (prescription and treatment). It is being interpreted as something totally different from what the yogis intended. The yogis believed the energetic channels must work together and be balanced and cleared in order for the kundalini energy to ascend from the base of the spine to the crown, producing enlightenment. Instead, today it is seen on prescriptions as if saying, "Here, take this drug. It's going to make you feel really, really good. It's going to change your brain waves. It's going to make you feel more aligned with who you really are."

The question is "Do we really need to take drugs to feel better?" Perhaps, in certain situations that is true. However, I believe that we can, for the most part, find different, non-drug solutions, like yoga. Let's analyze the caduceus from a Kundalini Yoga standpoint.

Kundalini Yoga identifies energy channels for the flow of consciousness. These energy channels, called *nadis*, seem to correspond to the meridians of traditional Chinese medicine. The 72,000 or more such channels or *nadis* are thought to carry the life force energy, known as *prana*. These *nadis* connect at special points of intensity known as *chakras*.

Each of the major chakras is associated with a gland and major nerve plexus that controls the area of the physical body in which it is found. For example, the Root Chakra is located at the base of the spine and is responsible for our sex organs and organs of elimination.

Just like negative and positive charges of electricity flow through a circuit, energy flows throughout the body the same way. As it flows through the *nadis*, the energy affects the chakras. One's overall health corresponds to how positively his or her energy field vibrates. Energy field disturbances can be seen as distortions of the chakras.

The 72,000 *nadis* arise at the navel point and end in the palms of our hands and soles of our feet. This is one reason why the "core" or navel point is an important focus for treatment in therapeutic rehabilitation. Interestingly enough, yoga practitioners typically do not wear shoes, so that all 72,000 *nadis* can be activated. Furthermore, in reflexology, a healing modality in which the total body is reflected in the hands and feet, the simple massaging of one's hand or foot can sometimes rehabilitate a particular body part that has been hurting or causing issues.

Of the 72,000 *nadis*, 72 of them are vital, and three of these 72 are of utmost importance. They are the *ida*, the *pingala*, and the *sushumna*. Reflecting back on the caduceus sign, the left side of the winding snake is the *ida*, the right side is the *pingala*, and the *sushumna* is in the center. The *sushumna nadi* begins at the base of the spine where the Root Chakra lies. The *ida (apana)* on the left represents the negatively charged feminine energy or the lunar or moon energy, which has a calming and cooling effect on the body. *Apana* refers to the eliminating functions of the body. Through exhalation and retention, the *apana* is drawn upward from the Root Chakra to the navel point. The *pingala* on the right (*prana*) carries the positively charged masculine energy, or sun energy, which has an energizing and awakening effect on the body. Through inhalation and retention, *prana* is directed down to the navel chakra or core area from the base of the heart and the neck. Thus, the *ida* and *pingala* unite and meet at the navel point, which starts to stir up and ignite the energy at the base of the spine.

The *sushumna* then lights up, causing the two polarities to raise the Kundalini energy. Often referred to as the Silver Cord, the *sushumna* then ascends. The *ida* and *pingala* travel only the distance between the nose and the base of the spine. That is why nasal breathing is essential for keeping the body balanced and strong (Bhajan Y. Prana, vayus, nadis & Kundalini. [lecture transcribed] 1/1/1976. Yogi Bhajan Lecture Archive).

This swirling energy continues its journey from the base of the spine to the top of the head, opening all the chakras along its pathway. Once it reaches the top of the head or the Crown Chakra, awareness and consciousness change. Going back to the caduceus, the wings represent the feeling of being awake and alive, feeling light and airy within the mind and body.

It is important to remember that the Kundalini energy lies inactive until the *ida* and *pingala* energies merge. During the Kundalini journey, lower body energy or vibration can be transmuted into higher forms. Healing can occur in areas that have been blocked for many years. For example, an individual with a jaw problem like temporomandibular pain (TMJ) might simply need pelvic floor work in order for his or her jaw to be restored to health.

How can our brainwave patterns be altered? When the Kundalini heat rises the pineal gland, also known as the seat of the soul, transmits a beam of energy toward the pituitary gland, thus opening the Third Eye and subsequently opening the Crown Chakra. Yogis believe that when the Kundalini heat rises this causes the energy of the glandular system to combine with the energy of the nervous system, leading one to total awareness. As this happens, the mind flows, awakens, and moves into an alpha brainwave state (daydreaming with eyes open, but still aware).

Kundalini yoga is a technology. The practice of yoga offers tools to set off this amazing energy. The purpose of Kundalini energy is to circulate the *prana*, which is done through breathing exercises that help activate the diaphragm and navel point. The breath is the most essential act, not only in yoga but also in life – because without breath, there is no life. Mudra*s* or hand positions are also used to activate the 72,000 *nadis*. Other tools used in Kundalini Yoga are the postures or asanas, eye focus, locks (a way of closing off a section of the interior body) and mantras or chanting.

For health professionals, it is important to teach yogic postures for rehabilitation that focus on the core connection to the diaphragm, the transversus abdominis, the pelvic floor, and the lumbar multifidi. Our future as professionals will require us to teach our clients to breathe correctly (from the nose) and to incorporate the breath along with exercise. By emphasizing the breath, our clients will heal more quickly because the Kundalini energy will be better able to circulate throughout the entire body. In addition, using different points of eye focus can help clients see themselves better internally, release any fears of performance anxiety, and rely more on their own internal body cues and instincts. Better yet, using sound with our clients as a sensory modality and also for those with visual impairments can help enhance functionality.

I hope you are able to see how a systems model can be a successful approach to care. Having an understanding of various modalities which can be integrated for treatment and how they overlap in philosophy can also be beneficial to your understanding of health and wellness. Now it is time to share with you how your anatomical systems all connect, just like the modalities.

In Chapter 10, you will see how these modalities or tools can be combined or used separately both as preventive measures and as creative treatment ideas for some health issues.

Chapter 10: Are You Breathing Correctly?

"Lack of activity destroys the good condition of every human being, while movement and methodical physical
exercise save it and preserve it."
Plato

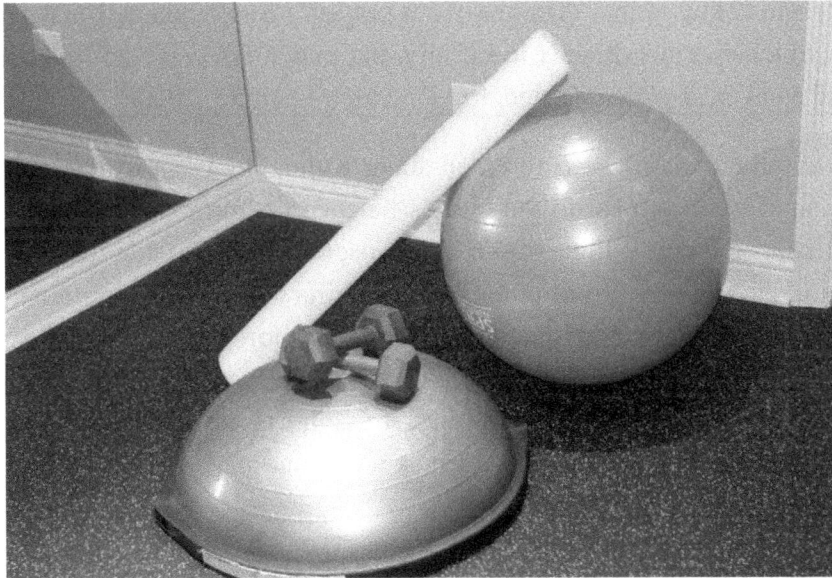

Have you ever heard idioms like "a breath of fresh air," "catching one's breath," "gasping for breath," "take a deep breath," or "under one's breath"? There are many more idioms about the breath. It is unfortunate that most of our society doesn't really understood how to breathe and the importance of the breath, nor do they take the time to be aware of the breath.

I was in Thailand in 2008. I remember waking up almost every morning to the chanting of the monks. Their sounds filled the air like a sweet lullaby. At that time, I did not know what the sounds meant, but my friend, a yogic teacher who accompanied me to Thailand, explained that they were meditating. It was strange to me that these remarkably powerful sounds were emitted from a very distant place at such an early part of the morning. It was even before the sun had made its beautiful entrance into the sky. I was fascinated by this amazing routine that took place every morning.

My friend asked me, "Do you know what meditation is?"

I responded "Not really."

She spent part of the early morning explaining that meditation is when the mind becomes completely clean and open so that infinity can communicate with you. Using what she had learned through her Kundalini yoga training, she described it as a two level process by which the self, meaning you, talks to infinity, and infinity talks back to the self or you. She went on to discuss how this process can resolve conflicts, and one can reach a state of shuniva – a state of absolute stillness where you become without thought and void of fears, the ego, and judgment. You become nonreactive to any situation or conflict.

I questioned then, "How is that different from prayer?" She explained that prayer is more one-sided by which you talk directly to infinity, but may not receive an immediate response that is felt and awakened within. (Kundalini Research Institute, 2010).

She went on to tell me that there is research about Kundalini Yoga which validates that the hours before sunrise are critical to the body's balance of hormones and neurotransmitters which are influenced by the pituitary gland. Neuroscientists claim that these early hours are when the endocrine and neurotransmitter balance shifts from relative domination by sleep-inducing melatonin to relative domination by serotonin, norepinephrine, and cortisol. If this shift doesn't occur smoothly, it can have a disastrous effect, like leaving you groggy all day, or it can cause overproduction of the stress hormone cortisol, which can create agitation and immune dysfunction. It can make you age early. (Khalsa, D.S., Stauth, C, 2001).

After she had reported this research, it all became very clear to me that instead of getting up and running to my local coffee shop for a boost to start my day, it would be better for me to sit like the monks and actually become high on life with the added benefits of improving the health and wellness of my body. So now, even the idiom "take a deep breath" has a new, deeper meaning.

Exercises Using the Breath of Fire

Completely understanding the breath or prana can really connect everyone as **one**, just like all the monks' voices became **one**. Let's learn some new ways to breathe and become aware of the breath. We will apply the breath to exercise, and then learn how to apply the breath and exercise into meditation.

Set a timer and start off slowly with the exercises. Increase your time once you have mastered each one. Any of these exercises can be done throughout the day – anytime, and anywhere.

By this time, you should be aware of the importance of conscious breathing and have learned how the diaphragm works and how to properly inhale and exhale. You should also be aware of your breath during every precious moment of your life. Practicing breathing exercises, as you will soon see, lowers your respiratory rate, improves your vital capacity – the amount of forcibly expelled from the lungs after a maximum inspiration – develops your cognitive functioning, and increases the ability to hold your breath for longer periods. Breathing exercises can even lower the amount of dangerous free radicals and increase the body's antioxidants. (Kupnik, D, 2003).

Long deep breathing or using the full capacity of the lungs will lead to increased endurance and patience. When you emphasize inhaling, the sympathetic part of the Autonomic Nervous System improves the heart rate, blood pressure, and your overall alertness. Similarly, emphasizing exhaling activates the parasympathetic part of the Autonomic Nervous System which slows the heartbeat and circulation and calms the nerves, relaxing our overall body, mentally and physically. If the breath is less than 4 breaths per minute, the pineal gland starts functioning fully and deep meditation becomes automatic. (Bhajan, Y, 2007).

When you are doing long deep breathing, think about inhaling health, strength, faith, peace, love, compassion and positive energy, and exhaling disease, weakness, fatigue, fear, tension, and judgment. Imagine yourself like a butterfly, able to fly freely through the skies without any restraints of life holding you back.

In the past, many people have asked me about being able to breathe in through your nose and out through your mouth. For people with respiratory diseases, breathing in and out of the nose may be a challenge. An alternative is to do pursed-lip breathing. Pursed-lip breathing causes air to become trapped in your lungs, helping to get more air out and making breathing easier. This technique is often used for those who may have asthma. Simply inhale through your nose and exhale through pursed lips, or exhale as though you were going to whistle. Be sure to exhale two times more than you inhale. (Fren, R, 2012).

When you begin breath work, just like any other exercise program, it is important that you consult a medical practitioner. Breath of Fire, the breathing exercise that I will describe shortly, should not be performed by pregnant woman or a woman during her menses. I tell my clients who have a heart condition or kidney condition to avoid Breath of Fire exercises. Children should not perform Breath of Fire until after the age of five.

It's a very powerful breath exercise, and if performed for three minutes, it could help to re-circulate your blood. Yogi Bhajan provides an excellent summary of the benefits of the Breath of Fire:

- Strengthens the navel chakra.
- Increases physical endurance.
- Strengthens the nervous system to resist stress.
- Expands the lung capacity and increases vital strength.
- Repairs the balance between the PNS (Peripheral Nervous system) and SNS (Sympathetic Nervous System).
- Reduces addictive impulses for drugs, smoking, and bad foods.
- Adjusts electromagnetic field.
- Boosts the immune system and helps prevent diseases.
- Stimulates splanchnic nerves in abdominal cavity, potentiating release of stimulating epinephrine and norepinephrine
- Produces an alpha and beta wave condition in the brain, creating increased calmness and heightened alertness.
- Increases oxygen delivery to the brain, creating a focused, intelligent, and neutral state of mind.
- Synchronizes the biorhythms of the body systems (Bhajan, Yogi. 2007)

Let me share a funny story showing how powerful this breath can be. In 2009, I went to India on a Yogic retreat. At that time, I was a competitive runner who was training for some ultra-marathons. I was extremely regimented with my training and running schedule. My biggest concern about leaving the United States was would I be able to run in India or even have time to run.

When I arrived in India, I was alarmed by the pollution and the lack of space for any type of running. In addition, my schedule was quite packed with learning meditation and yoga. My teacher could see my worry and disappointment. She approached me in a quiet moment away from the others and told me that I would stay in the same physical shape and have the same strength and endurance when I returned to the United States. She just explained that training was going to be done in a different way and that she would help coach me through it.

My training as I soon found out was to do Breath of Fire for fifteen minutes a day for the entire month there. And sure enough, I returned back to the United States stronger both physically and mentally. My endurance even improved.

If you know you are a paradoxical breather and don't understand the biomechanics of breathing, then Breath of Fire is the perfect place to learn. Just by undertaking this breathing exercise, your navel center will naturally and automatically move toward the spine on exhalation.

The easiest way to teach this exercise is using the breath through the mouth. However, the goal is for you to perform the exercise diffusing the breath in and out of the nose, the area in where the IDA and PINGALA meet, while keeping your lips gently closed.

An essential part of learning the Breath of Fire is that you follow all the body cues that I have given you in earlier chapters. If you have forgotten, then I will remind you. Your pelvis needs to be in neutral, your head in neck lock, your eyes closed, relaxed and focused on the third eye point, your jaw relaxed and dropped, your fourth and fifth digit squeezing to bring your shoulder blades back, and movement originating from the navel center. Please use these postural cues from now on for all of the breathing exercises, in all other exercises, and in the meditations.

Now that you are in perfect posture, let's begin. I want you to begin by sticking out your tongue and panting like a dog. You are probably thinking that you look funny. Don't worry about it. Just pant.

There should be a sound quality to the breath. Listen carefully. At first, the inhalation and exhalation may not sound equal. After you continue for 30 seconds, your breath should regulate itself and the sound quality of the inhalations to exhalations should match. Of course, everyone has their own rhythm in their body.

Think of it as similar to an athlete who is going out for a run. There is a time when this athlete must properly warm up by starting the run slowly in order to build up oxygen within his/her system. The runner's heart rate and breathing pattern may fluctuate until a plateau occurs where there is now flow and synchronization with all systems of the body. Don't be discouraged. My rhythm is always a little off at the start of this breath. Give yourself time to develop a tempo. It will get easier every time you begin Breath of Fire. You are just learning.

Breath of Fire – Panting like a dog

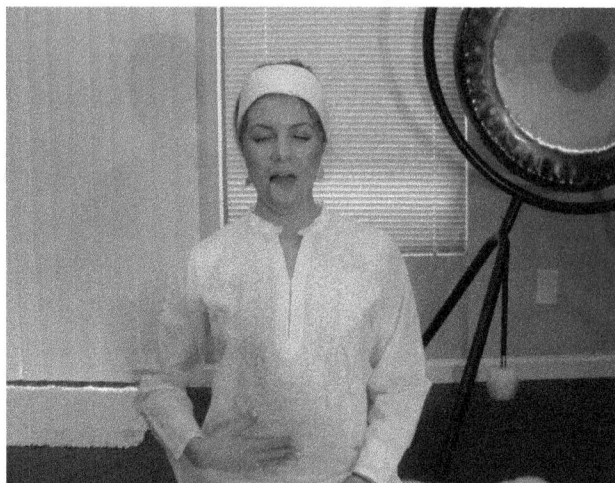

A little word of advice: please make sure you drink water while doing this breathing exercise. It is an intense exercise because you are basically detoxifying your body and re-circulating oxygen and blood throughout your body. It is normal to have a metallic taste on your tongue and dryness in your mouth. You are getting rid of toxins within your body. Your body is getting a massage through the breath work. Water will keep your body hydrated and refreshed.

You may even feel a little light-headed or dizzy. Your brain wave patterns may have switched to the alpha frequency and this may give explain your current state of mind. Don't panic. Drink water. You may even need to eat a little snack.

It is important to start off easy. As you understand the breath and feel connected with it, begin to increase the time and frequency of the breath. I like to give my clients or students a set time to perform the Breath of Fire. This is called a time-contingent approach.

For example, I may say, "Continue the breath for three minutes." I'll give them motivation and cues along the way until they reach this time frame. Often, when we are struggling with an exercise or activity we do not feel comfortable with, we will just give up. Most likely, that is because our mind has expectations which cause our bodies to just quit. Remember, focusing fully on the breath will keep your mind and body working together and block all your negative self-talk.

So, read this paragraph and then close your eyes. Sit up straight. Do the Breath of Fire for approximately one minute. Use a timer if you are doing this by yourself. When you are ready, you will set a timer and begin. Listen to your panting sounds. Focus on the breath.

Go within. Inhale, suspend the breath. When the timer rings, take a deep breath. Hold it. Fill your abdominal area, your chest area and your neck area. Hold it there. Hold it there. Then exhale.

When you feel complete, you can slowly open your eyes. Powerful? Hot? A little dizzy? Do you have that metallic taste in their mouth or any dryness?

The reason that I ask you to suspend your breath is because I am challenging you to build up your system's endurance in order to improve your sympathetic nervous system. The result can be to breathe fewer breaths per minute. When you to suspend the breath and hold it there, you literally take in more oxygen to fill all the different areas of your body and let the oxygen begin saturating these areas. Holding the breath allows you to create a new set point as to how much oxygen you can take in over a period of time. When you exhale slowly, you're influencing your parasympathetic nervous system by relaxing the body and creating homeostasis. It is also a great way to get rid of a headache or sinus infection.

Now that you have mastered Breath of Fire through the mouth, it is time to do it in and out of your nose. This could be challenging at first, but it is similar to mouth breathing. Give your body time to adjust to this breath. Begin the Breath of Fire through the nasal passages with the lips gently closed. Set a timer and try to accomplish this breath for one minute. You should really feel the navel pumping and the spinal muscles being activated.

The best way I can describe doing breath of fire through the nose is the action of doing forceful sniffs through your nose. A good visual guide is that you are pushing air out as if you are fogging up a mirror. The breath should never be forced. Listen to the sound of the breath. It is okay to increase your rhythm and tempo when you feel that you have connected with your breath.

When I give lectures and teach this breath, I always ask for a volunteer who has a fear of speaking in front of an audience to come up to the front of my class. I invite the volunteer to briefly tell the class about themselves and what prompted them to attend my class. I ask the class to observe the volunteer as he or she is speaking. My hope is that the class evaluates tone of voice, eye contact, body and hand positioning, and comfort level speaking.

After the brief introduction, I have the volunteer remain in front of the class and perform Breath of Fire for one minute with the entire class. Once this is completed, I then ask the volunteer to retell her story about herself. Usually, the class is instantly surprised, as is the volunteer speaking. There are multiple changes between the first and second speech. After the Breath of Fire exercise, the volunteer will usually feel more grounded which is reflected in his/her stance and body positioning. There is better eye contact, a more controlled tone of voice, more animation and fluency in his/ her voice, more hand gestures and movement, and overall, more comfort and ease with speaking.

The Breath of Fire really helps activate the navel center. In fact, singers are taught to sing from the navel center. The navel center helps produce a grounded tone and more overall oxygenation to hold a tone.

Try singing a song and listen to your voice. Then do Breath of Fire, sing again and listen to your voice. Did you hear the difference? I often will make it a point within my day to do some Breaths of Fire, especially in between seeing each of my clients. It really helps me gain some extra energy and clear my head so I can become more present.

Using the One Minute Breath

I'd like to introduce another breathing exercise called one-minute breath. It involves inhaling for 20 seconds, holding the breath for 20 seconds, and exhaling for 20 seconds. This breath is excellent to get rid of confusion. It helps with focus and centering and changing a negative thought into a positive one.

If you are just learning how to breathe from your diaphragm, this breath exercise can seem challenging. So, I advise my clients to start with inhaling for 5 seconds, holding the breath for 5 seconds, and exhaling for 5 seconds, eventually building up to the 20 seconds. As with any new exercise, it takes time to get your body in a rhythm. This breath will help improve both the parasympathetic and sympathetic nervous system and lower your heart rate and blood pressure.

You can imagine that as your inhaling, you are climbing a ladder from the navel center to the top of the head and climbing back down on exhalation. This breath requires opening up each energy center and filling your body with an abundance of oxygen; holding the oxygen so it can circulate; and then cleansing all the body and ridding of it of toxins upon exhalation. You will feel more balanced.

If you can, do a five or ten-second breath. You can mentally count, "one, two, three, four, five," or you can use your fingers to count to stay engaged.

Now you try it. Either do the five-second breath or the ten-second breath. Before you begin, don't forget those postural cues. By the way if you would rather lie on your stomach or back to do this breath, it is okay. Find a position that is comfortable for you.

Let's turn now, your attention to nasal breathing. Do you remember that in Chapter 9, I wrote about the yogic channels, and I mentioned that the left channel is called the Ida and the right side is the Pingala. The Ida and Pingala come together or merge at the navel center, move through the chakras, and intersect at the nasal passageways.

Each of these energy channels has a different function. The left side is moon, feminine energy that is cooling and calming .The right side is sun or masculine energy known for its fire and activity. Breathing in and out of the left nostril can help with relaxation and sleep and calms the nervous system. On the other hand, breathing in and out of the right nostril can help activate the sympathetic nervous system and can give you lots of energy.

For example, people who suffer from having a deviated septum and breathe mainly through the right nostril will have problems with blood pressure. A simple operation to correct this problem can help equalize the breath in both nostrils and normalize blood pressure (Kupnik, D, 2003).

Previously in this book, I spoke about the importance of nasal breathing from a medical standpoint. Now, we can understand it from a yogic viewpoint.

I'd like to discuss the diagnosis again of paradoxical vocal-cord dysfunction. Speech therapists are now treating individuals with this diagnosis by focusing their treatments on nasal breathing. Individuals with this diagnosis are usually performance-driven athletes. They get so caught up in their athletic activity that they may hyperventilate or acquire acid reflux type symptoms. When respiration is normal, the vocal cords are supposed to partially abduct or spread apart with inhalation. Instead what happens is the vocal cords adduct, come together, upon inhalation, causing the closing of the airway passages, hyperventilation or pH changes to occur within the brain. This, of course, is the opposite of what should happen during the respiratory cycle.

Treating hyperventilation is simple. People treat hyperventilation by covering their mouth with a bag and blowing into the bag. The best treatment is closing your mouth and gently breathing in and out of your nose. This will automatically rebalance the pH levels within the brain.

Nasal breathing is also the best way to relieve sinus infections and headaches. In fact, according to EEG recordings, higher activity of the right brain hemisphere results in easier breathing through the left nostril and higher activity of the left brain hemisphere results in easier breathing through the right nostril. This cycle fluctuates every 25 to 200 minutes. (Kupnik, D, 2003).

Let's practice nasal breathing. Begin by placing your thumb up against the right nostril with the other four fingers extending up toward the ceiling. Keep your head in neck lock and follow all the postural cues. Hold the right nostril gently and breathe in and out of the left nostril. Close your eyes and focus on the third eye point. Begin conscious breathing for one minute.

Listen to the sound quality of this breath. It will sound as if you are surrendering air out of the nose. Focus on creating a letting go, relaxing, reducing air sound. This will help with anxiety, hypertension (high blood pressure), hypertonicity (increased muscle tension), and it can actually lower blood pressure and heart rate. If people with sleep disorders can sleep on their right side, they will compress the right nostril, causing them to breathe in and out of their left nostril. This stimulates the left brain hemisphere and improves the parasympathetic nervous system.

Now switch hands and do left nostril breathing. Place your thumb up against the left nostril with the other four fingers extending up toward the ceiling. Keep your head in neck lock and follow all the postural cues. Hold the left nostril gently and breathe in and out of the right nostril. Close your eyes, focus on the third eye point, and begin conscious breathing for one minute. Listen to the sound quality of this breath. It should be a sniffing sound as if you are trying to get air up and into all parts of your body. This breath is good for motivation and extra energy. It can to relieve depression and assist with sports performance. It also is beneficial for clients with hypotonicity or generalized weakness. It stimulates the right brain hemisphere and improves the sympathetic nervous system. Heart rate will accelerate, and blood pressure will increase (Bhajan, Y, 2007).

Right Nasal Breathing

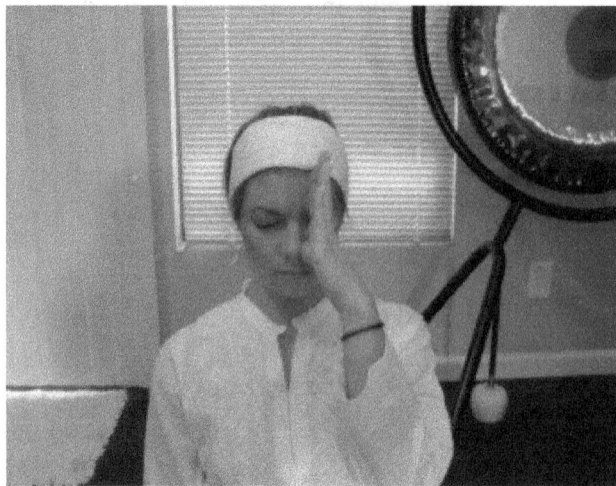

Congratulations on learning these breathing exercises. If you still have not mastered conscious breathing or the basics, then this next section is for you. I have found that the majority of my clients are unaware that they are breathing incorrectly. If I ask them to practice any sort of home program or exercise, they will either start to turn red in the face – and that is when I know they are forgetting to breathe – or else they just don't understand how to exercise and breathe at the same time. Often these clients complain that there is too much to focus on. Guess what? If you don't breathe correctly when exercising, you will have difficulty healing and getting rid of pain. Your constant complaining about a problem will not end it. The breath or pranayama is as necessary as the physical exercise. The two must co-exist for healing.

It is important to remember that any breathing exercise can be done in any position. You can teach the following exercises in supine or on your back, prone or on your stomach, or even sideline. I often will put a client in sideline to help eliminate gravitational forces. For example, if a client just had shoulder surgery and was unable to lift his/her arm up to the sky, I would place them in sideline which would eliminate the gravitational pull on the arm and allow for successful range of motion. In the following exercises, I will specify a position, but remember it is okay to think outside the box.

Most yoga classes teach the relaxation portion in the supine position or lying on your back. These poses are actually considered the most important part of the class. Relaxation helps center one's emotional energies, releases stress, relaxes tight muscles, improves blood flow, revitalizes the parasympathetic nervous system, creates vibration throughout your body, and helps release old habits. The supine position is an excellent position because it gives your body proprioceptive input from the ground. The ground forces are able to give your body immediate feedback about where your body is in space and about pressure, balance and coordination. This position will also increase the supply of oxygen to the body and allow you to exhale larger quantities of carbon dioxide produced during exercising.

Relaxation Posture – Supine position

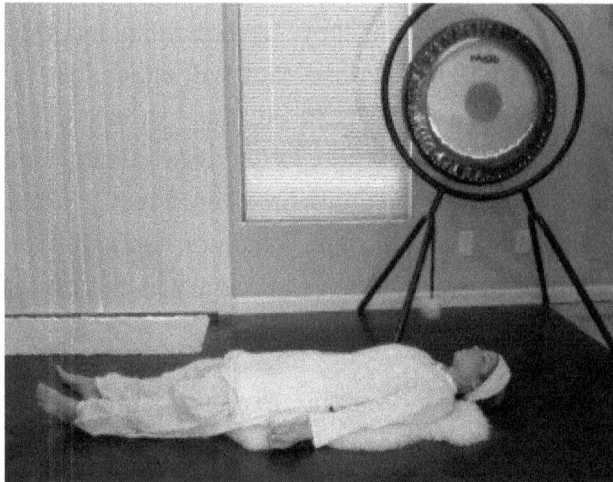

Ovarian Breathing

Ovarian Breathing is a very special exercise that really reiterates diaphragmatic breathing. I learned this breathing technique during a birthing course, *Birthing from Within*, created by Pam England. You can use this breath during birth or any time to help quiet the mind and refocus on the breath. It also helps direct your breathing to the correct process of inhalation and exhalation.

To perform this activity, you will need a partner. Once you have mastered this breath, you can do it alone by imagining that a partner is present, assisting you. I often seat a client on a chair in proper alignment so their feet are flat on the floor.

I begin by placing the palm of my hand on their sacrum area. As I tell the client to inhale, I move my hand up from the sacrum to the crown of the head, resting it lightly on the top of the head. The client is instructed that as my hand moves up from the sacrum to the top of the head, he or she is to inhale through the nose or fill the body up with air at each segment that my hand is gently touching. (Inhale. Inhale. Inhale.) The navel center should move out and the chest, the neck and head areas should expand with air in proper diaphragmatic breathing. I often have the client imagine that his/her energy channels are being opened up as my hand moves up toward the spine.

There is a pause at the crown of the head between the inhalation and exhalation phase. It is important to note that you can either perform this activity by gently placing your hand on your partner's back or just using the heat of your hand to deliver tactile cues.

As the client exhales, I will move my other hand down from the crown of the head to the pubic bone. My hand will not be touching the client's body but the heat of my hand will guide the exhalation phase. The client will slowly exhale through the nose from the top of the head slowly to the pubic bone. The client's breath on exhalation should be felt on my hand as I continue to move my hand down from the top of the head to the pubic bone. (Exhale Exhale, Exhale) I observe and the client understands that air is exhaled segmentally from the head and neck area to the chest area to the navel center, eventually forcing that center to move in toward the spine.

One of my hands should always remain in contact with the body; one on sacrum during inhale and on crown during exhale, while other hand moves with the breath. Eventually, the client can close his/her eyes while doing this breath. Verbal cues are given by me throughout the process and eventually lessoned as the client masters the breath. This exercise can be done in sideline. Remember to always ask permission whether it is okay to touch someone's back while you are performing this or any exercise.

Ovarian Breathing Inhale/Exhale

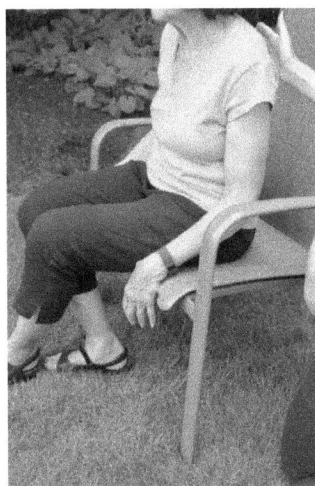

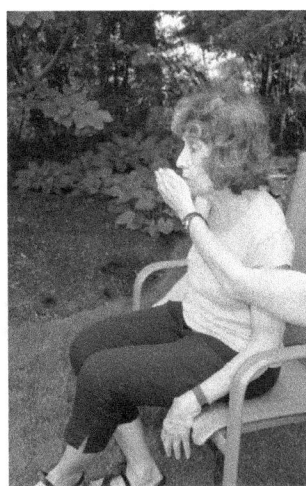

Birthday Candles

This breathing technique called "Birthday Candles" is often done with a partner. The purpose of this technique is to help a partner or client who is having issues with diaphragmatic breathing to experience the sensation of the breath through the other person's body. Two people will lie on the floor on their backs. The individual having difficulty understanding diaphragmatic breathing will lay his/her head on the other person's navel center, using the other person's navel center almost as a pillow. The person who understands the process will then begin proper diaphragmatic breathing.

As this person inhales, his or her navel center will rise giving immediate feedback to the individual whose head is on his/her navel center. This feedback will continue as the person using proper diaphragmatic breathing expands during inhalation and releases the breath upon exhalation, breathing in and out of the nasal passageways. The individual resting on the other person's navel center will follow the rhythm of the other person. By doing this, not only will they learn to sense each body segment inhaling and exhaling, but they will also be able to successfully mimic the process breathing in and out of the nasal passageways.

Both individuals may keep their eyes closed during this breath. Continue doing this breath until both people are in rhythm and have become skilled at the breath.

Birthday Candles

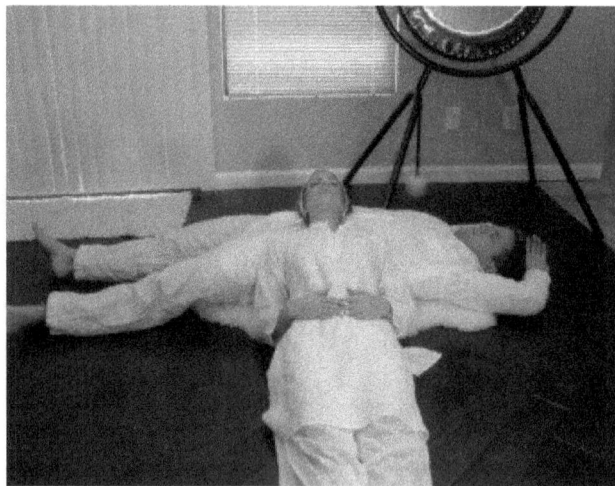

Hockey Puck, Beanie Baby Breath and String Techniques

Hockey Puck or Beanie Baby Breath is a great exercise to really implement all parts of segmental breathing/diaphragmatic breathing. You practice filling up your body with as much oxygen as possible upon inhalation and release toxins upon exhalation. You also learn how to not cheat the breath or use assessor muscles. This breath can be used to teach any type of client, (geriatric, pregnancy, and back patients) or any individual not identifying with diaphragmatic breathing.

Ask the client lie on his or her back on the ground which provides great proprioceptive feedback. Continue with postural cues and have the client keep the eyes open at first and then close his/her eyes when the breath is done correctly. Place beanie babies, hock pucks or objects that will give good tactile feedback on the client's navel center, chest area, and neck or clavicular area. Tell the client to begin breathing. You may also give feedback using your hand in addition to the object.

Have the client inhale. As they inhale through the nose, make sure the client is seeing or feeling the object move up toward the sky. With each inhalation, the puck or other object should be seen moving up correctly, beginning from the navel center and upward with each segment of breath. On exhalation, the objects will be seen or felt to lower down as the client exhales from the top of the head, to the chest, to the navel center.

Beanie Baby Breathing

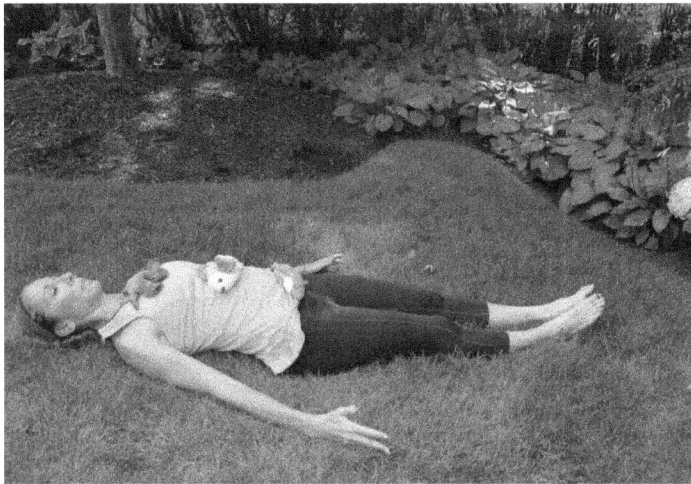

String is another tool that you can use if you're teaching clients how to perform diaphragmatic breathing while sitting. Have the client place a string around his/her navel center. Have them hold it firmly around this area. Follow all the postural cues before beginning the breath.

Instruct the client that upon inhalation, the navel center should push out and make the string become tighter and on exhalation the navel center should move toward the spine, making the string become looser, decreasing the space between the string and the navel center. You can use a belt, string, or even yarn.

Prone over Swiss Ball or Prone on Elbows Breathing Exercises

Now that you have gotten the hang of diaphragmatic breathing, let's try a different position. Being on your belly, either on the floor or on a Swiss ball should offer you both tactile cuing and immediate feedback. That is of course, if you are performing diaphragmatic breathing correctly.

While on your stomach, inhale pushing the navel center into the ground or ball. Inhale segmentally in and out of your nose until you get the breath to the head and neck area. On exhalation, feel your navel center move back toward the spine. Exhale in and out of the nose from the top of the head to the navel or sacrum area. Make sure you follow the postural cues and close your eyes to really become linked to your body.

Prone on elbow breathing

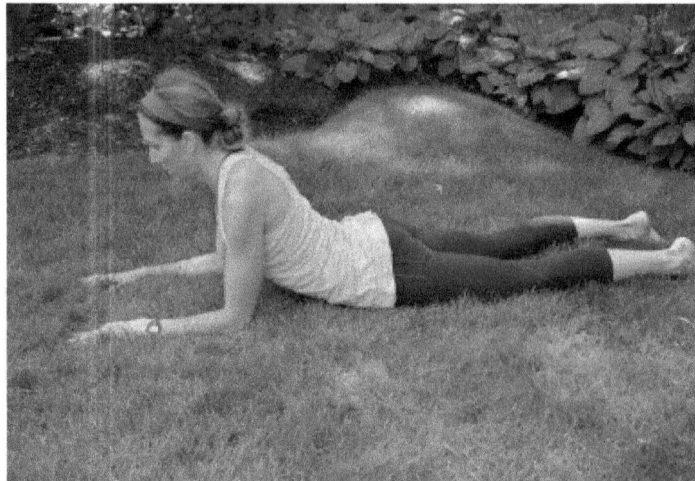

Prone over Swiss Ball

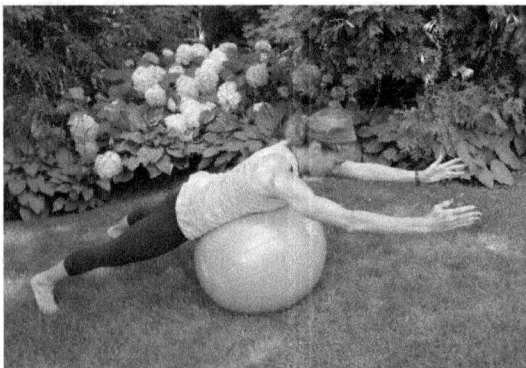

Kneeling over Swiss Ball

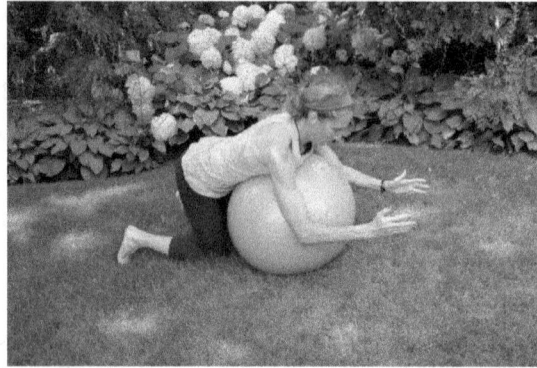

Supine Positions

For this position, I'm going to ask you to lie on your back and raise your arms straight up to the ceiling with your thumbs up and other fingers fisted. Slowly bring your arms down. Please follow all the postural cues and breathe in and out of your nose. As you raise your arms up, you are going to inhale segmentally, moving the navel center out and expanding the chest and neck area. Just by raising your arms up with your fingers fisted, you should automatically feel that you are diaphragmatically breathing.

Now, slowly exhale, bringing your arms back toward your chest and keeping your hands fisted, feeling the navel center move toward your spine. Continue doing this exercise until you can really feel the breath incorporated with the movement.

Once you feel comfortable with this movement, now switch and hold onto a Swiss ball and perform this exercise. Inhale while lifting the Swiss ball toward the ceiling. Then exhale while lowering the Swiss ball down toward your body.

You can also try this exercise on your side. Remember to relax your neck and keep your spine straight with your knees slightly bent. If you are trying to get more stretching in your right arm then position yourself on your left side and for stretching more of your left arm, position yourself on your right side. Simply inhale and move the ball out in front of you; then exhale, bringing the Swiss ball back toward your body. The great thing about this exercise is you can vary the angles that the ball is moved out in front of your body on the inhalation. Challenge yourself so the ball can be maneuvered toward your other shoulder or down toward your hip.

Supine with Swiss Ball – Inhale/Exhale

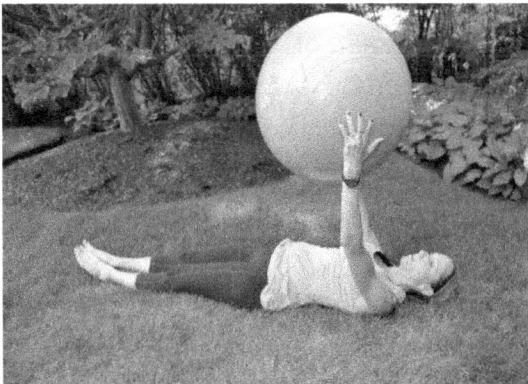

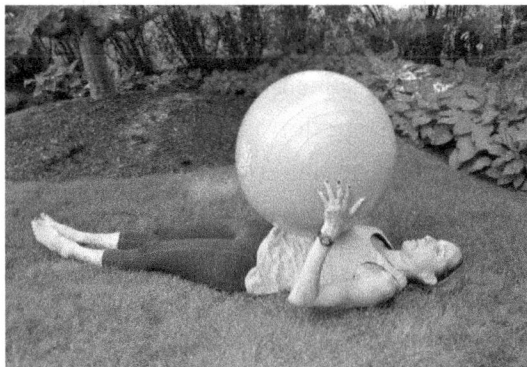

Sideline – Inhale /Exhale

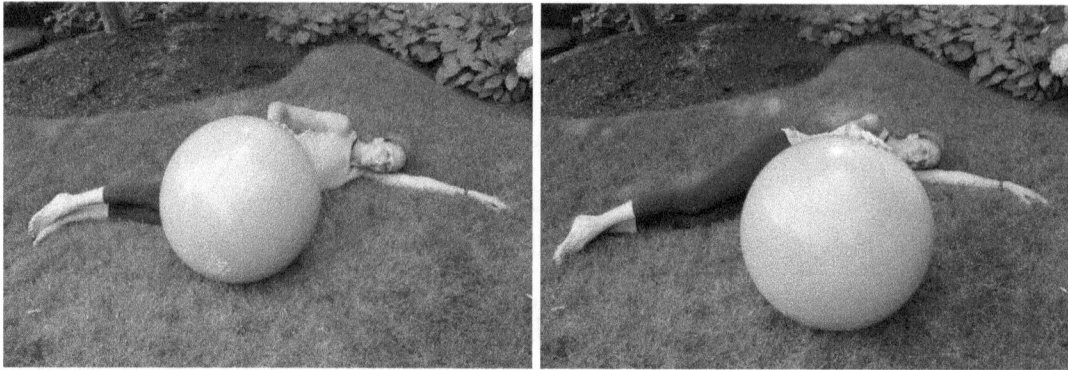

Washing Windows

You can do the Washing Windows exercise by yourself or with an individual who has problems with diaphragmatic breathing. If this is done in sideline or in sitting position by yourself, place your hands on a wall as if you are washing the wall.

This is a great exercise because it not only teaches clients how to breathe, but it also improves their trunk control for rolling, bed mobility skills, shoulder range of motion and even transfer training, such as sit to stand. I will often sit in easy pose, Indian style. If you choose this position, please make sure that you are in good postural alignment. Remember that it is okay to place a pillow underneath your fanny to bring your pelvis more into an anterior pelvic tilt.

I will first teach you how to do this with a client. For example, a client of mine has shoulder issues from a recent right shoulder surgery and lacks range of motion within her right shoulder. At the same time, she is unable to breathe correctly. I have found that often when I ask a client to perform a movement, they will have performance anxiety, and with this comes fear and breath-holding. An easy way to help clients overcome this is to have them close their eyes. This will automatically bring their focus inside and help with breathing.

As a therapist, I'm going to play an active role in her therapy session. I will begin by placing my palms up against the palms of her hands. Sitting in good postural alignment on chairs, we will both be breathing in and out of our noses. I will first guide her through a movement pattern using my arms and breath. My sound quality will be exaggerated so that she can mimic the breath with the movement. It is kind of like a dance. I will be leader first and then I will have her take over the dance and lead me.

The goal is using diaphragmatic breathing with movement. So, if my arms go up, then I will inhale and when my arms are brought down, I will exhale. This active, assisted range of motion can be done in any plane of movement so long as the breath is incorporated correctly. After one minute, I will switch roles and have her lead me. I may decide then to have both of us move into the sideline position and perform this movement. Again, I will lead and she will follow and then vice versa. This is an exercise she can learn to execute on her own using a wall, only then she is in charge (Khalsa, S. K., 1998).

Washing Windows in Easy Pose

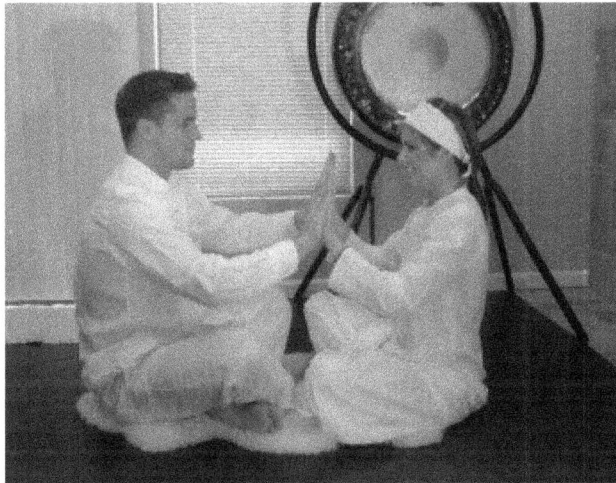

Row, Row Your Boat

This breathing/movement exercise is designed to teach diaphragmatic breathing and moving from the navel center. It will help with transfer training (sit to stand or bringing your nose toward your toes). It can be performed in any position and can even be done with or without a partner.

If done independently, I will often tie an exercise resistance band to a doorknob. Next, I sit in a chair in good postural alignment, holding onto the Thera band with both arms. Like "Row, row, your boat," I will inhale, rocking my pelvis forward, moving from the navel center and pulling the Thera band back, squeezing my shoulder blades together. On exhalation, I will rock my pelvis backwards, moving from the navel center, and releasing the Thera band back to normal.

If I choose to do this with a partner, I will sit in a chair across from my partner. Both of us will have our arms crisscrossed. One person will rock forward as the other person rocks backwards. Each of us will be breathing correctly and moving from the navel center. There should be no poor posture observed because the movement will be directed from the navel center. You may do this with eyes open or closed. Remember, closing your eyes will provide flow and uninhibited movement (Khalsa, S. K., 1998).

Row, Row, Row Your Boat in Easy Pose

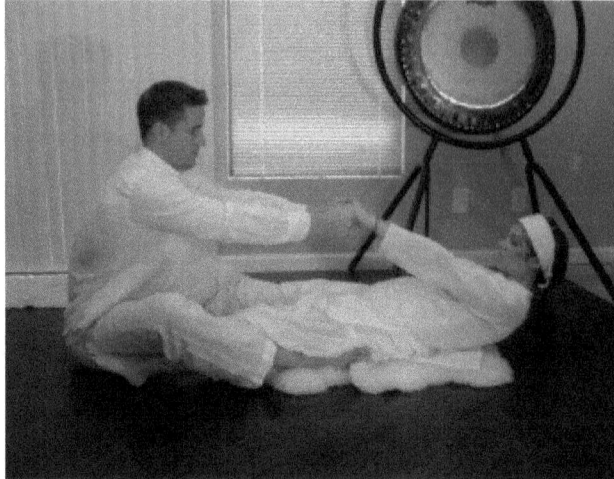

Congratulations on learning to take the time to breathe correctly. Now that you have successfully achieved the breath in different positions and understand the dynamics of breathing, it is time to enhance your life by using the breath with all kinds of exercise. Now that you know how to do it effectively, take a deep breath!

Chapter 11: Combining Breathing and Calisthenics

"Without proper breathing, the yoga postures are nothing more than calisthenics."
Rachel Schaeffer

Do you remember when you were in gym class in grade school and high school? Prior to playing or doing a sports activity, the teacher would require some form of warm-up or calisthenics. Calisthenics is a form of exercise intended to increase body strength, body fitness, and flexibility. These exercises were also supposed to loosen the muscles and help with focusing. But did they really?

Recall whether you did those exercises with much awareness and if you were even moving from the navel point? I bet you were flailing your body every which way and seeing how fast you could do the exercises so that you could move on to the planned sport activity? Did the teacher or instructor just stand in front of the class and blow the whistle when time was up? Was his or her instruction limited to "Give me 10 jumping jacks?"

I can guarantee that you weren't thinking about the core connection or compressing your diaphragm with each exercise. You probably did not have much brain/body connection using sensory input either. As far as incorporating the breath with the exercise, I doubt that probably ever took place.

In the pages to follow, I will be explaining the Do's and Don'ts of each callisthenic exercise or yogic exercise that you will recall doing in grade school or high school. These are very standard exercises given to clients today within my physical therapy practice. I think everyone will remember and relate to these exercises.

Can you imagine what the difference will be when performing these exercises the correct way? There are several key points to remember when performing these exercises:

- Relax your eyes;
- Drop your jaw;
- Squeeze your fourth and fifth digit together to bring the scapula into retraction;
- Squeeze the shoulder blades together so the diaphragm opens;
- Keep your pelvis in neutral, not slouching, so that you have an equal base of support with your feet;

- Avoid standing on the inside of your feet;
- Keep your head in neck lock;
- Keep your pelvis in root lock.
- Make sure you use your breath -- inhale and exhale.

For example, if you are flexing your arms or bringing your arms up to the sky, make sure you keep your thumbs up so the ball and socket of the shoulder joint can rotate and allow for movement above ninety degrees. If you raise your arms with your thumbs down at ninety degrees, the ball and socket joint will have difficulty rotating and the nerves can be pinched between the joints. Inhale when you are bringing your arms up to the sky and exhale when you bring your arms back down to your sides.

The following exercises can be done with added equipment like weights, the Swiss ball, a foam roller and so on. You may wish to alter the position of the exercise, like performing an exercise on your side instead of in sitting. This can reduce the impact of gravity so that it will be easier to lift your arm or leg. For example, with the spinal flex exercise, you may have difficulty focusing on your diaphragmatic connection when sitting. Perhaps lying on your side when doing the exercise will not only help ground your pelvis and give you good proprioceptive input, but will also reduce the influence of gravity.

Try to remember to use nasal breathing, move from your navel point, and use sensory input to connect with your body (vision, sound, touch, smell). Close your eyes and go within to remove any ego and any judgments you may have about your body. Feel and sense who you truly are at your core. The yogic postures found in this chapter can also be found in Yogi Bhajan's book, *The Aquarian Teacher* (Bhajan, Y., 2007).

You may want to take off your shoes and socks and begin to wake up all your energy centers by rubbing the palms of the hands and the soles of the feet together. Also, you may want to dim the lights and add some aromatherapy. I like to take an orange and cut it in half and squeeze it around the room. This helps me awaken and helps my creative juices flow. I also use lavender to help relax me and help me focus better. Let the tension GO! Good luck!

Improper Shoulder Flexion   Proper Shoulder Flexion

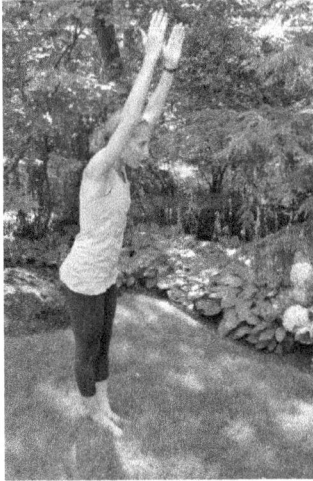

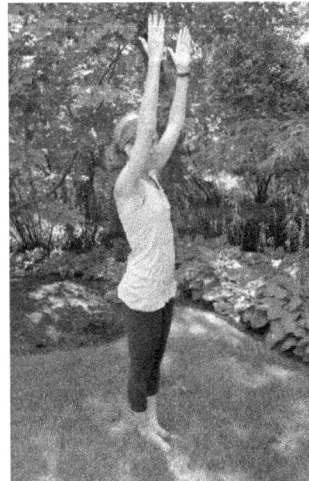

Now we are going to practice. I'd like you to get on a mat or sit in easy pose or sit on a chair. Choose whatever you feel is more comfortable so that you can really sit upright and so that the pelvis is open. Try and use all the postural cues and diaphragmatic breathing skills as you just were taught. Start performing each exercise within this chapter for 30 seconds and then progress as needed.

Spinal Flexion and Extension Exercises

I mentioned earlier about Michael Gach. If you remember, he always does two things as part of his daily routine: he rubs his ears and he does what's called Spinal Flexion and Extension Exercises to open all his back meridians.

With Spinal Flexion, the movement is always going to come from the navel center. Sit in easy pose or sit in good postural alignment. Close your eyes. You're going to inhale. You will rock the pelvis forward, but as you do, you're going to move from the navel center. You will be opening up and expanding the chest upon inhalation. On exhalation, rock the pelvis back. Try as hard as you can to stay still and not collapse the navel center. The movement is at the navel center itself and everything else stays steady. There should be no slouching.

Try this for 30 seconds. You might feel like you're starting to shake. Don't panic. This just means you're reawakening your nervous system.

Improper Spinal flexion/extension – inhale/exhale

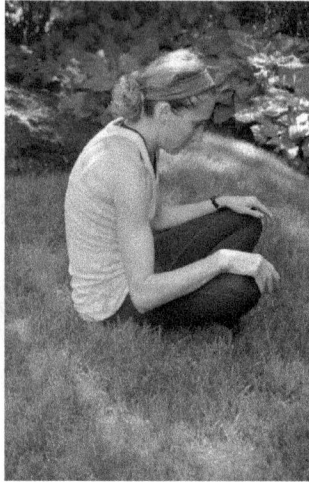

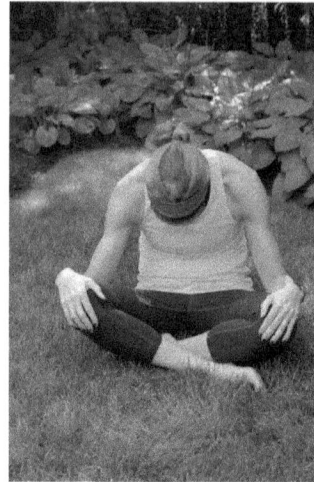

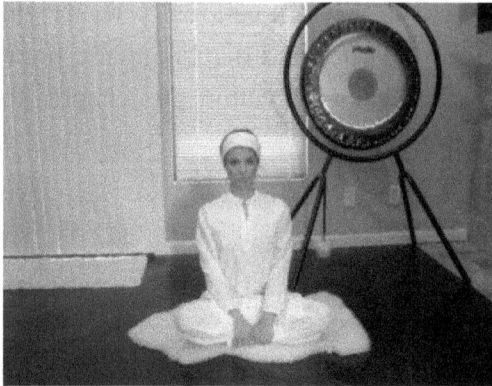

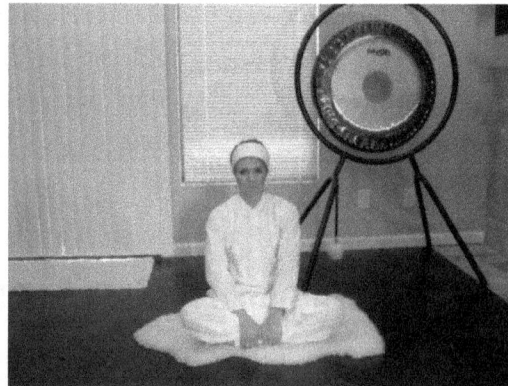

Proper Spinal flexion/extension-inhale/exhale

Sufi Grinds

Now, let's do what is called "Sufi grinds." They are very similar to trunk rotations where you sit on a Swiss ball and do circles on the Swiss ball. However, most people who get on the Swiss ball and do trunk rotations are bending from their waist and have no connection to their breath. The idea behind Sufi grinds is to open up the pelvic floor, which will help with digestion and any issue connected with the pelvic floor.

Visualize that there is a circle underneath your behind, and you're going to draw the circle using your pelvis. Sit either on a chair, in easy pose, or on a Swiss Ball. The movement will come from the navel center. Avoid collapsing. You must use the breath with the movement.

For example, Mr. Jones, a client of mine has left-sided weakness. He is always sitting on his right side and neglecting any movements to the left side. What I tell Mr. Jones when he is doing this exercise is to emphasize making circles with his pelvis, directed toward his left side. By doing this exercise, anyone will discover imbalances or postural habits that need correction.

Imagine a clock. Move your pelvis to the right and hold the inhale from 12 until 6. Then exhale to the left side from 6 to 12. If a client has difficulty holding the breath for that long, break down the clock into shorter inspirations and expirations. You can also reverse and start inhaling to the left and exhaling to the right side. Placing a clock in front of you as a visual aid will help.

Proper way to perform Sufi Grinds

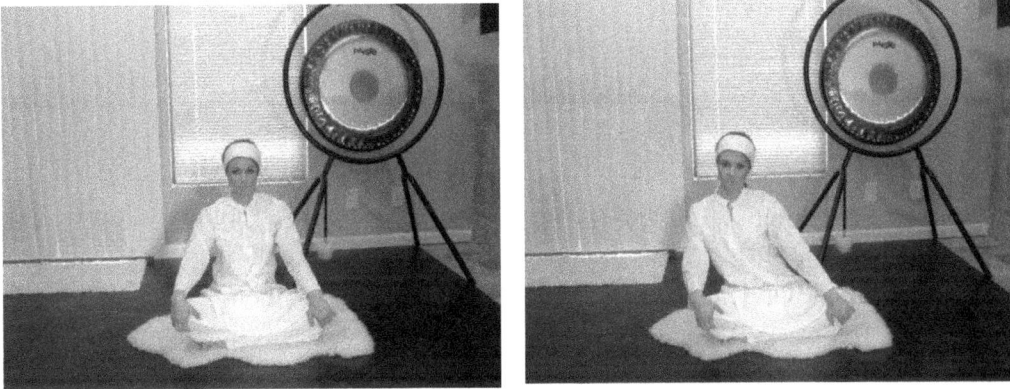

Improper way to perform Sufi Grinds

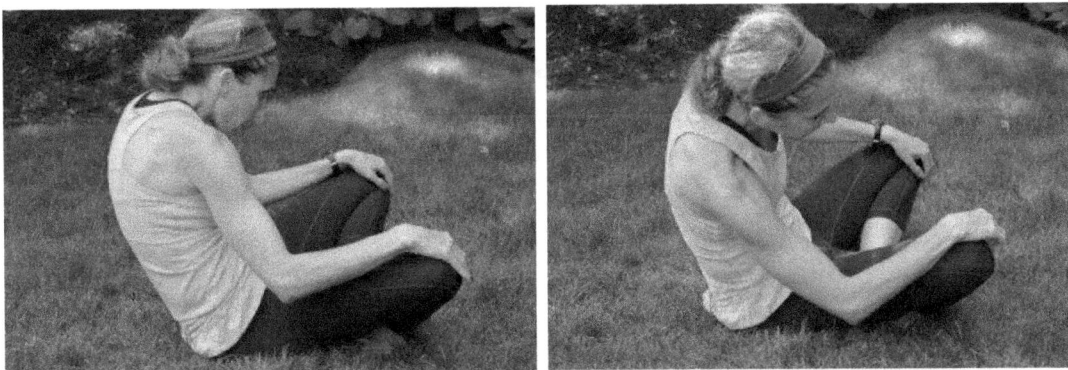

Sufi Grinds on the Swiss ball in proper alignment

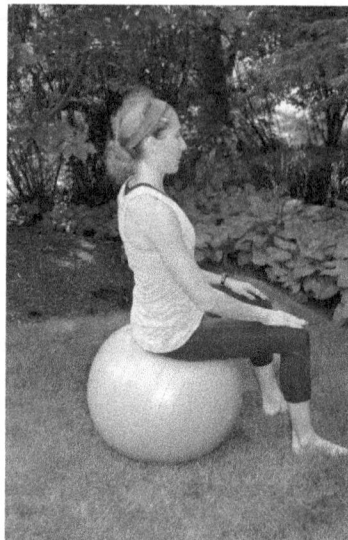

Shoulder Shrugs

Let's try shoulder shrugs. Sit on a chair or on the floor in easy pose. Sit in good postural alignment and breathe in and out of your nose. Keep your spine straight and move from the navel center. Inhale and bring your shoulders to your ears. Exhale bringing your shoulder back to neutral. Inhale and imagine your body is filling up with light, love, compassion, positive energy. Exhale and imagine you are getting rid of negativity and things that no longer serve you.

Proper Shoulder Shrugs

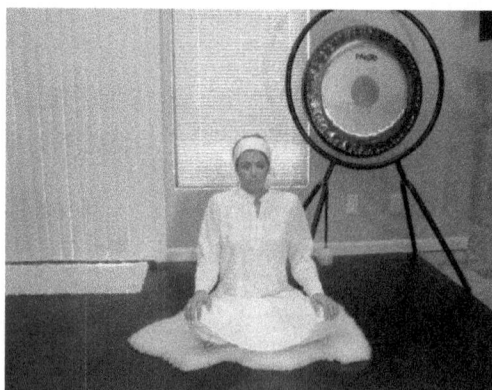

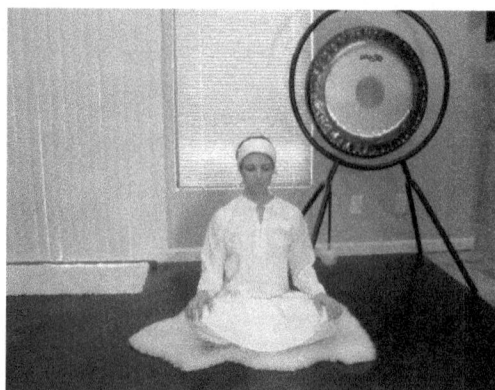

Improper Shoulder Shrugs

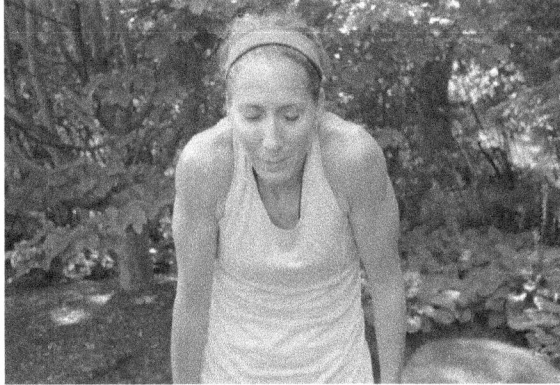

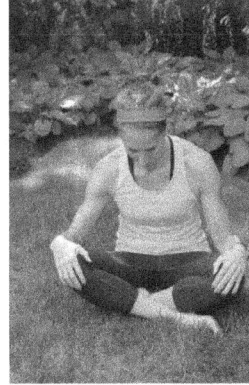

Neck Rolls

Neck rolls are very similar to Sufi grinds. When you are asked to do neck rolls, be careful not drop your neck too far forward. When our neck goes forward, our shoulders want to go forward also, and then our diaphragm gets compressed.

You're now going to visualize that all of your movement will originate from C7 vertebrae (the 7th cervical vertebrae of your cervical spine). This is the hump or vertebrae prominens which sticks out from the back of your neck. It is a fulcrum point and all movement must come from this point.

Just as you did with Sufi grinds, you are going to get in a position and visualize inhaling to the right from 12 to 6 o'clock, and then from 6 o'clock all the way back to 12 o'clock using your C7 point. You can reverse this and inhale/exhale to the left. When you come to center with your head, you're not really dropping your head forward, but keeping your head in neck lock. If you drop your head too far forward then your shoulders may round and your diaphragm may become tight.

Proper Neck Rolls

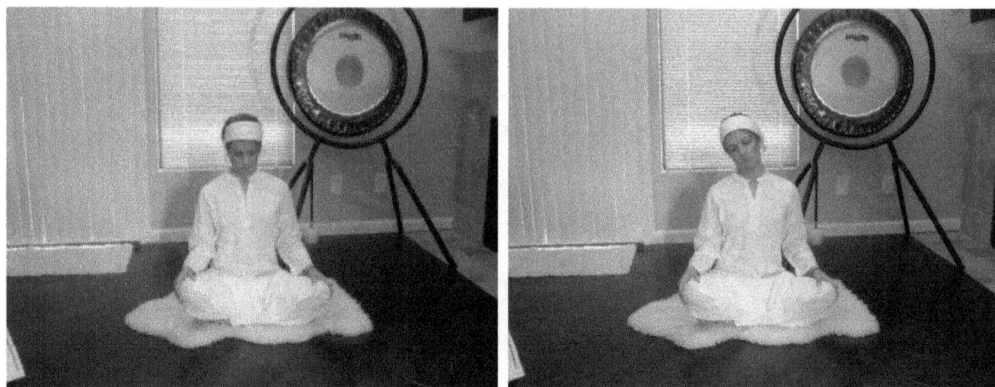

Improper Neck Rolls

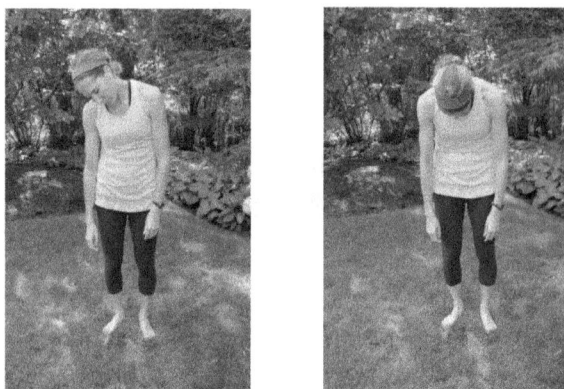

Straight Leg Raises

Begin doing straight leg raises by lying on your back. In yogic practice, we have what is called angles and triangles. Raising your leg to different levels will affect different energy systems in your body. When you bring your leg about six inches off the ground and then bring it down, this stimulates the reproductive system. Notice whether you are in control or are you just whipping your leg up and down?

Now, you are going to change the quality of movement. First, place your pelvis into root lock. Squeeze your rectum and your sex organs and bring your navel towards your spine. Holding root lock lift your right leg off the ground, but incorporate an inhalation as you raise it up. Then bring the leg down as you exhale. In other words, you're going to inhale up and then exhale down, but you're going to still hold root lock.

Continue doing the right leg for three repetitions. Then work with the left leg, performing three repetitions. Do you notice more control with your legs? It might seem a little bit more difficult, but the benefit is that you're actually working the muscles, the circulatory system and the respiratory system and having a conscious connection to the exercise that you're performing.

Proper versus Improper Straight leg raises
90 degree angle/lift both legs and just one leg.

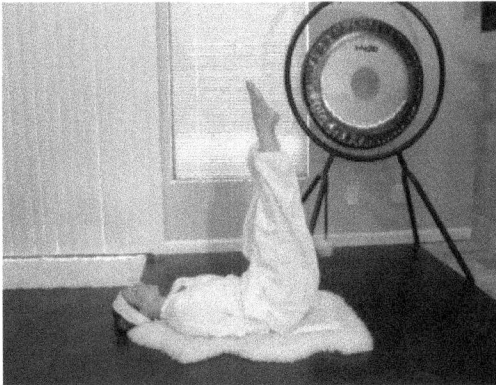

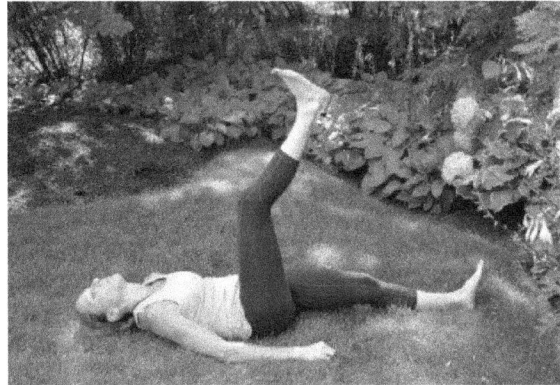

Bridging/ Pelvic Lifts/Hip-Ups Exercise

The Bridging/ Pelvic lifts/Hip-ups Exercise_is one of my favorite exercises. I will often include this exercise as part of a home exercise program for my clients. I see most of my clients just lifting their buttocks up and down with no conscious connection to the breath or to their body when they initially perform this exercise.

To do this exercise correctly, before beginning you must apply root lock which grounds the pelvis to the floor. You are going to hold root lock and inhale slowly visualizing that as you are lifting your behind, each part of the spine from the navel center to the head area is being lifted, segment by segment. Your chest will expand and your heart center will open.

Now exhale, but instead of just plopping your buttocks down, you're going to visualize that as you're exhaling, you will lower your spine segmentally from the head all the way to the tailbone area. The tailbone will be the last segment to touch the ground.

When you do the exercise in this way, you may experience a Kundalini awakening, during which your nervous system is firing and the pelvis is awakened, activated and sending out electrical signals. Your legs may start to shake, but just place a pillow between your legs for support. Modifications for this exercise include keeping your arms at your side or under your buttocks to support your back. If you are more advanced, you can hold your ankles.

Proper and improper way of performing bridging/pelvic lifts/hip ups exercise

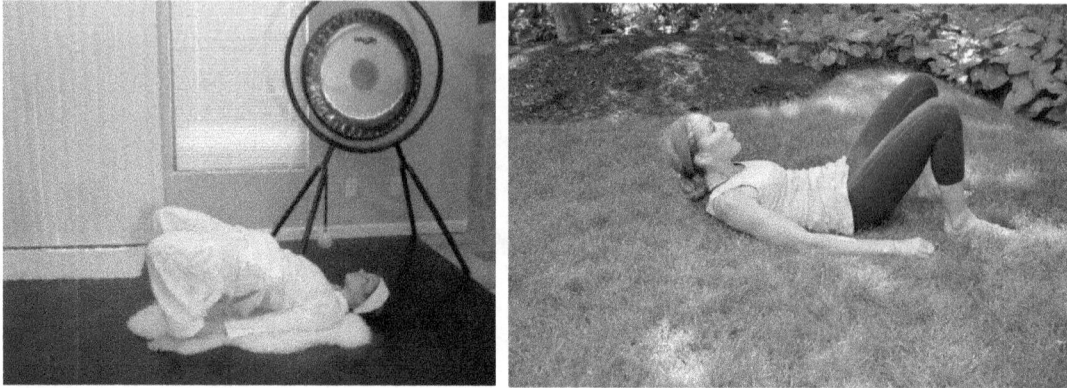

Proper Ways of Doing Familiar Exercises

Here are some other improper versus proper ways of doing some common exercises!

Tree Pose- improper versus proper way

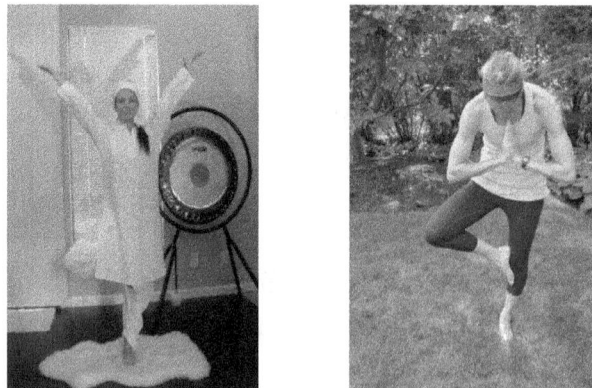

Spinal Twist -Improper versus Proper

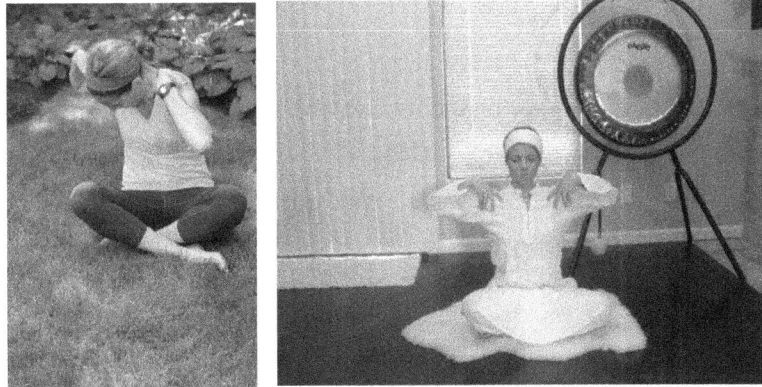

Reaching for your toes: Improper versus Proper Way

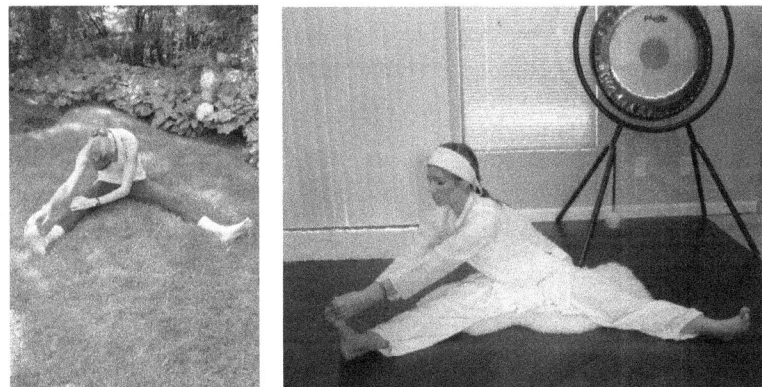

Have you ever heard someone say, "Go and meditate!?" I was very confused when I first was told to go and meditate. I didn't know what that meant. I thought, "Okay, I will go and sit and breathe." However, I discovered that doing only that was ineffective since I didn't know how to breathe properly and I was easily distracted by my surroundings.

Did you know mediation is an art form? It can involve many components. Meditating can really help your mind develop patience and give it a road map to follow. It is often the mind that steers us away from our directional path. In fact, there have been studies demonstrating that meditation results in enhanced attentional performance and fewer oversights in tests of visual attention.

Of course, we need the physical body to work alongside the mind for cleansing, tuning, and repairing. Once the mind and body become one, the art of meditation is achieved. In the same way that playing many instruments in an orchestra together can produce a beautiful melody, your being can vibrate a new sense of self and awareness.

During meditation, your eye focus may change, your breathing rate may alter, your hand positions may be different, your body positions may shift, and you may even want to chant like the monks. Each meditation is different and requires, at first, some concentration and practice. Learning meditation is just like acquiring any new skill in life. It is similar to going to the gym to build your muscles, but you can do meditation almost anywhere, and the benefit is that you can build your body's overall health.

I ask one thing as you learn the following meditations, and that is that you aren't critical of yourself. Give yourself time to learn this art.

Speaking of time, Yogi Bhajan made it clear that each minute of meditation had some effect on the body and mind. He said, "Three minutes of meditation will affect your electromagnetic filed, your circulation, and stability of the blood. Eleven minutes can change your nervous system and glands. Twenty-two minutes balances your three minds, positive, negative, and neutral, and they begin to work together. Thirty-one minutes allows the glands, breath, and concentration to affect all the cells and rhythms of the body. Sixty-two minutes changes the gray matter of the brain, and two and a half hours can change your psychic, magnetic field and create subconscious new patterns." (Bhajan, Yogi, 2007).

It is important to not forget the precious moments in our life. As you breathe and meditate more, you will discover that things will actually get done much faster and with greater ease. Don't sit and stress out over little things. Get going and learn to meditate. Here are three easy meditations that you can give to yourself as a gift to be done every day.

Focusing on Your Pulse

An easy way to begin to learn how to meditate is to sit in easy pose and place your eye focus on the third eye. Place any four fingers of the right hand on the left wrist area, feeling the pulse. Do not place your thumb on this area because your thumb has its own pulse. Focusing on your pulse will help you to concentrate better and bring direction to a wandering mind. Focus on the breath.

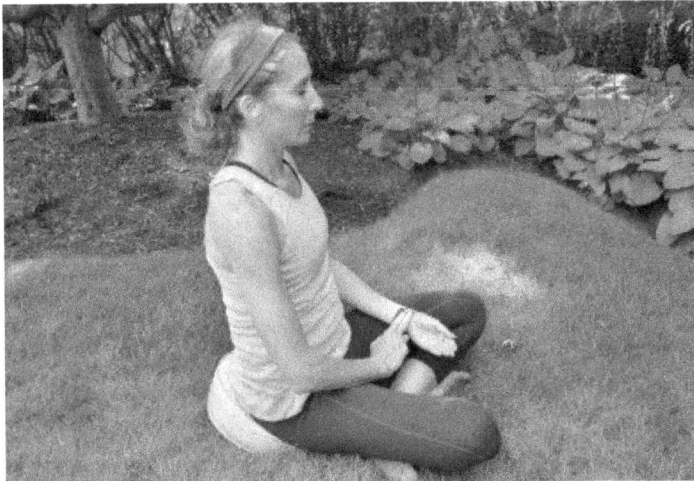

Breathe for Energy

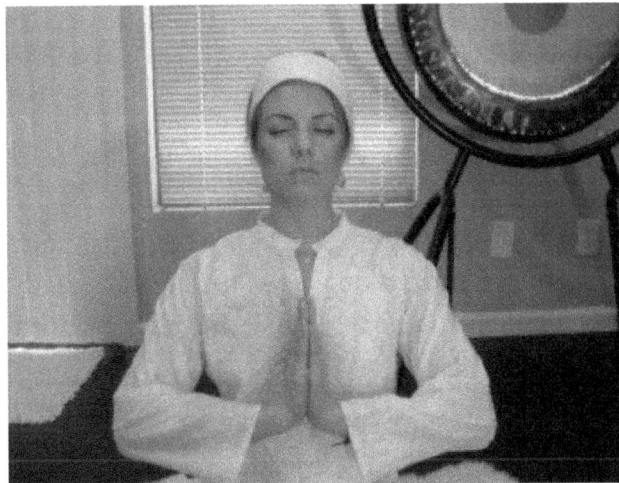

- Sit with spine straight in a chair or in easy pose.
- Palms are together at the heart center in prayer pose with thumbs pressed against the sternum.
- Focus between the eyebrows, with eyelids slightly closed.
- Inhale through the nose in equal parts (like sniffs). Exhale in 4 equal parts. On each sniff, powerfully pull in the navel.
- Continue for 3-5 minutes
- End by inhaling deeply and press palms together with maximum force for 10 seconds. Then exhale and relax for 15-20 seconds. Repeat this 2 more times. (Khalsa, M.K., 2008).

This meditation helps overcome anxiety, confusion, and commotions of the mind. Through awareness of our breath, we connect with our inner selves. We may begin to experience a power bigger than ourselves. It keeps our mind in a positive state.

Meditation for the Negative Mind

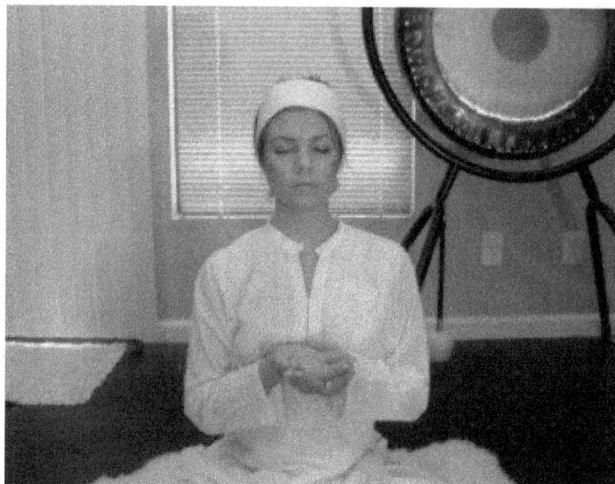

- Make a cup of the hands with both palms facing up. The right hand rests on top of the left.
- Place the cup at the heart center. Elbows are relaxed at the sides.
- Eyes are slightly open and looking down towards the hands.
- Inhale deeply through the nose. Exhale through rounded lips. Feel breath on your hands.
- As you inhale, allow unwanted desires or negative thoughts to enter your mind. As you exhale, completely let them go.
- Time-11 minutes
- At the end of the meditation, inhale powerfully, and exhale completely through the nose. Repeat this breath 3 to 5 times. Then relax completely.
  (Khalsa, M.K., 2008).

This meditation helps to ward off negativity. It clears the mind of unwanted negative or fearful thoughts, protecting and enhancing our livelihood.

I hope you have been able to witness how the calisthenics exercises we learned in school are very similar to yogic postures. The difference is in our alignment or posture while we are doing the exercises and in the way we breathe. Furthermore, now if someone asks you how to meditate, you will have an answer and can even give a demonstration. It is that simple. Our posture and our breath play a significant role in almost everything we do every day. Let's now learn how to come up with preventive ideas for some well-known ailments.

Chapter 12: How to Think Outside the Box for Ideas of Some Medical Ailments

"Continuously learning and improving is the only way to grow. Continuous learning helps fully develop natural abilities and creates a curious, innovative mind."
Dr. Anil Kr Sinha

Congratulations for making it this far in this book. It is now time to integrate all the knowledge that you have read. Hopefully you have learned and understand some alternative methods to treat yourself or someone else who may have the following ailments:

- Back pain,
- Temporal mandibular or jaw joint disease,
- Hypertonicity (tonal issues -- highly muscular),
- Pelvic floor issues,
- Neck pain,
- Acid reflux,
- Scoliosis,
- Balance and coordination problems,
- Paradoxical vocal cord dysfunction,
- Asthma, and
- Hyperventilation.

The goal of this chapter is twofold. It is designed is to give ideas of how to think outside of the box, allowing you to be more creative in your approach to healing. Also, it will assist you to use the systems model approach, challenging you to look deeper into the cause of a problem before making an assumption or judgment. You can apply both of these approaches to each of the above problems. After you have read each treatment, I encourage you think of other ideas that you might wish to add?

Thinking outside the box is an important tool to acquire. I remember my interview with one of the physical therapy programs to which I applied. As part of the process, I was asked to sit in a room and choose one of ten societal issues currently being debated. I was given only ten minutes to come up with pros and cons to the issues. Then, I was placed in front of a panel of therapists to debate my points. Of course, throughout my debate time, I was barraged with lots of questions and clarifications.

Looking back on the day of the interview, I felt unprepared and, of course, nervous. Today, I commend the school's program for putting me through such a strenuous process because it taught me so many valuable tools. I learned how to "think fast on my feet" because as physical therapists, we are required to evaluate our clients and come up with an immediate treatment plan. We also must be able to collect and analyze data and to come up with clear and rational solutions to clients' problems based on that data, research and our own clinical experience.

Ideas for Alternative Home Remedies

Below is a list of ideas that I gathered from all the chapters of the book. The treatment alternatives are categorized by ailment. These concepts can be used to help alleviate a possible ailment or problem that you may be experiencing. Each of the chapters that you have already read contained some vital information about posture, breath, color, vision, emotional ways to heal, and body awareness. They also described the influence of other modalities such as Reiki, acupressure, and yoga as well as the techniques of mapping the body's connections and core stabilization.

Now it is time to see how the information you have learned in each of the chapters can be coordinated into a program to help correct or heal a bodily issue. Realize that the organization of the ideas listed below is just a way my mind has selected to place each of these concepts. Your mind may think a little differently. The approaches below can be used in a preventative fashion as well as a remedial one.

Please make sure you or your client consult your doctor prior to trying any of these ideas if there is a risk of a health issue. Except when another author is cited, all chapter references refer to this book.

Let's begin . . .

Back Pain

- What are you holding onto? From Louise Hay, Chapter 5
- Fascial lines-superficial back line – Chapter 9
- Diaphragmatic breath-activation of diaphragm, TA or pelvic girdle, multifidus or muscle band attaching to the spine, and pelvic floor – Chapter 3
- Aromatherapy for relaxation (Frankincense to help slow respiration and regulate breath and Lavender) – Chapter 4

- Postural exercises-sitting, standing, walking – Chapters 4, 6, and 7
- Change in habits-work or functional Chapter 4
- Is extension of spine occurring with inhalation? Chapter 2
- Reflexology/Acupressure points (CV 6 or Sea of Energy, B 54 or Commanding Middle) with breath – Chapter 9
- Back rolls- using above acupressure points – Chapter 9
- Yogic exercises incorporating breath with movement - basic spinal flex, leg lifts, baby pose, windmill – Chapters 10, 11
- Wear blue glasses to calm nervous system – Chapter 7
- Tapping for muscle activations – Chapter 4
- Use of sounds for TA (pelvic girdle) activation-SSS, SHH – Chapter 3
- Always think navel toward spine – Chapter 2
- Which other muscles are tight which causes stress on the back? Chapters 3, 9
- Breathing exercises – Chapters 10 and 11
- Matching- move from internal structure – Chapter 4
- String exercise: put string around navel point, inhale navel point moves into string, making string tight; exhale, navel point moves away from string, string becomes loose – Chapter 10
- Reiki, a form of energy healing, using your hands – Chapter 8

TMJ- Temporal Mandibular Joint

- Change eye focus- relax eyes-loose jaw; eyestrain acupressure points; GV 25.4 or Third Eye point – Chapters 7 and 9
- Rub area around jaw - William Reich's work – Chapter 9
- Diaphragmatic breath work: make sure fill lungs and breathe in and out of nose, relax jaw or just breathing exercises – Chapters 2, 11
- Posture: forward head, slouching – Chapters 3 and 4
- Neck lock – Chapter 11
- Blue glasses – Chapter 7
- Light hands over area for Reiki or myofascial release – Chapter 8
- Release of abdominals, jaw point, inside of knee or iliopsoas; pressure on points and breath or any muscle along deep core line or superficial back line
- Foot placement when walking – Chapter 9
- What are you holding on to? Anger? – Chapters 5 and 9
- Yogic exercises with focus on dropping jaw and head in neck lock – Chapters 7, 10, and 11
- Avoid bad habits; too much stress will lead to tight jaw – Chapters 4, 6, and 7
- Wear blue glasses – Chapter 7

- Aromatherapy for relaxation (chamomile for toothaches, lavender for headaches) – Chapter 4
- Acupuncture points: GB 20, Gate of Consciousness – Chapter 9
- Mantra or chant with focus on tongue hitting palate – Chapters 4 and 9

Pelvic Floor Issues

- Focus on Connective tissue attachments -- jaw, eyes, diaphragm, TA (transversus abdominus or pelvic girdle), multifidus – Chapters 3 and 9
- Diaphragmatic breathing; no chest breathing – Chapters 2, 10 and 11
- What are you afraid of? Abuse affects your root chakra (foundation) – Chapter 5
- Squatting-postural exercises – Chapters 4 and 7
- Using Sound for activation TA and thinking navel toward spine – Chapters 3, 4, and 7
- Mulbandh (Root Lock) exercises or stop the flow of urine – Chapters 3 and 7
- Acupressure points-for constipation: (Sea of Energy-CV 6) – Chapter 9
- Reflexology points-Lungs – Chapter 7
- Pregnancy exercises: see breathing exercises and squatting – Chapters 2 and 3
- Yogic postures with diaphragmatic breath – Chapters 10 and 11
- Eyes close/visualization exercises: think of pelvic floor like bee hive. As bees move, they push pelvic floor open – Chapter 7
- Sitting in alignment exercises, no slouching – Chapters 3 and 4
- Look at how you sit; work station, habits – Chapter 4
- Pelvic lift exercises focus on diaphragmatic breath – Chapter 11
- Breathing exercises – Chapters 10 and 11

Tonal Issues – High Tone

- Rood techniques- including swiping with elbow at 90 degrees to open hand – Chapter 4
- Positioning- position opposite of tonal positions – Chapters 4 and 7
- Reflexology- foot and hands at lung area – Chapter 7
- Quiet environment-calming/classical music-helps decrease tone and bring two hemispheres of brain together – Chapter 4
- Aromatherapy- Lavender, Sandalwood – Chapter 4
- Colored glasses and adaptive equipment – Chapter 7
- Tactile cues at diaphragm to assist diaphragmatic breath – Chapter 4

- Visual cues- client focused on breath to area and add auditory cues – Chapter 4
- Acupressure points: for anxiety, GV 24.5 or Third Eye Point; C V 17 or Sea of Tranquility; Points for asthma and breathing: K27, Elegant Mansion – Chapter 9
- Breathing exercises – Chapter 10
- Reiki – Chapter 8

Neck Pain

- Neck Lock – Chapter 11
- Diaphragmatic breath; C3, C4, C5 – Chapter 3
- Yogic postures with diaphragmatic breath; neck rolls – Chapters 10 and 11
- See TMJ section
- Eye focus – Chapters 6 and 7
- Healing Affirmations for Neck/Thyroid: What are you afraid to speak about? From Louise Hay – Chapter 5
- Postural corrections: Are you sitting, standing, and walking correctly? Chapters 2, 3,6, and 7
- Blue glasses – Chapter 7
- Supine exercises for breathing: feeling alignment of neck, breathing in and out of nose, and connective tissue (squeezing third/fourth digit for scapular retraction). Is breath moving to neck or may require taping or tactile cues at chest area – Chapter 10
- Acupressure points, GB 20 – Chapter 9
- Reflexology points: Base of fingers and toes – Chapter 7
- Aromatherapy: lavender – Chapter 4
- Breathing exercises and Breath for Energy Meditation – Chapters 10 and 11
- Reiki – Chapter 8

Acid Reflux – see definition Chapter Two

- Diaphragmatic breathing – Chapter 2
- Postural correction- opening up diaphragm – making sure getting extension with inhalation – Chapters 2 and 3,
- Aromatherapy- Peppermint, chamomile – Chapter 4
- Acupressure points – see pelvic floor – Chapter 9
- What are you afraid to digest? – Chapter 5
- Work pelvic floor, TA, and multifidus – Chapter 3

- Massage clockwise around abdominal area: yogic exercises with focus on diaphragmatic breathing – see *Itsy Bitsy Yoga Book*
- Breathing exercises – Chapters 10 and 11
- Reiki – Chapter 8

Scoliosis

- Is it structural or nonstructural? – Chapter 6
- See Back Pain section above
- See scoliosis positioning – Chapter 6
- Light gentle distraction: sideline and opening up curve – Chapters 4 and 6
- Focus is on diaphragmatic breath – Chapter 2
- Yogi postures focusing on opening up curvature by using breath; example: pelvic lift with pillow under the shoulder and side that is compressed – Chapters 6 and 11

Balance and Coordination Problems

- Focus on eyes-use weighted vest: see Vision Section – Chapters 4, 6, and 7
- Use colored glasses – Chapter 7
- Aromatherapy- Peppermint for vertigo – Chapter 4
- Yogic postures using diaphragmatic breath with root lock when needed – Chapters 7 and 11
- Proprioceptive and vestibular activities: doing activities with shoes off sends signals to inner ear – Chapter 4
- See back, neck, pelvic floor ideas above

Paradoxical Vocal Cord

- Focus is on nasal breathing/diaphragmatic breath so vocal cords can abducted during inhalation – Chapter 10
- Focus on good posture – Chapters 2,3,and 6
- See acid reflux ideas above
- What are you controlling? – Chapter 5
- Teach meditation for relaxation and visualization – Chapters 10 and 11
- Chanting – Chapters 4 and 7

Asthma

- Diaphragmatic breathing – Chapters 2, 3, and 10
- Focus on good posture – Chapters 2, 3,6 and 7
- See back, pelvic floor, and neck ideas above
- Mediation – Chapter 11
- Relaxation – Chapter 10
- Buteyko Breathing: similar to nose breathing with eyes closed and looking up, exhale slowly until you feel that there is no air left in your lungs; hold your breath as long as you can and return to gentle breathing
- Yogic postures with diaphragmatic breathing – Chapters 10 and 11
- Pursed lip breathing causes air to become trapped in your lungs, helping to get more air out and make breathing easier. Inhale through nose and exhale through pursed lips, or exhale as though you were going to whistle. Exhale 2x more than you inhale (Fren, R, 2012).

Hyperventilation

- See Asthma and paradoxical vocal cord section above
- Focus on good posture – Chapters 2, 3 and 6
- Focus is immediately on nasal breathing. Breathe in/out of nose to help rebalance PH levels in brain – Chapter 10
- Reiki – Chapter 8
- Nijmegen (Hyperventilation) Questionnaire: Includes primary guide to breathing training and gives a broad view of symptoms associated with dysfunctional breathing patterns. Symptoms include chest pain, blurred vision, tightness around mouth, and anxiety

So, how did you do? Were you able to recall the alternative methods suggested, or, if not, could you use the reference for each of the ideas under each ailment to locate the appropriate method? I will bet that you may even be able to think of many more concepts to add to the list now that you have gotten this far. If not, take your time and go back to each chapter and review. In time, all the pieces will fit together and you will have a better sense of the body and all its amazing connections and systems.

Conclusion

"An Ounce of Prevention is Worth a Pound of Cure"
Benjamin Franklin

As you can see we are constantly discovering new information about our bodies. Let's start with the heart. The heart is the most electromagnetic organ in the body. The heart is the physical center of the circulatory system, managing 75 trillion cells (Dale, C, 2009). Researchers found that the heart is composed of 60 to 65 percent neural tissue which helps us with memory, emotional processing, and sensory integration. Do you listen with your heart, the organ for emotional processing, or let your mind make your decisions? I would choose my heart now that I know the heart's power.

The circulatory system takes the deoxygenated blood and moves it through our heart to our lungs. The lungs can then bring the oxygenated blood back through the heart and to our body. The whole circulatory system also collects toxins for delivery to the lungs, liver, and kidneys for excretion.

The lungs cradle and cushion the heart. The two systems, as we know, work together. They control breath, alter our heart rate, and provide waste removal and oxygen for cells throughout the body.

Breathing helps create movement in the spine, linking the breath to our muscles, bones, connective tissue, and fascia. Our breathing can alter our brain wave patterns, and help with sound production or vocalization.

Our rate of breathing is even controlled by the medulla oblongata, the respiratory center of the brain. When we breathe, the respiratory system also pumps cerebral spinal fluid and lymphatic fluid. As the lymphatic system flushes from our system foreign bodies, chemicals, and bacteria, our immunity gets a boost. The breath gets rid of toxins through lymph nodes located in the groin, armpits, and neck. As we breathe correctly we may experience a bitter taste in our mouths and dryness. That's the lymphatic system at work. Any exercises that we do around our neck area, armpits, and hips will immediately affect our lymph nodes.

The Yogis always recognized the navel area, as the autonomic mesenteric nervous system. It has as many neurons as the spinal cord does, but distributes them diffusely over the abdominal area and intestines rather than consolidating them in a single tract. So by exercising and breathing correctly, the fire energy at the navel point will help with digestion, speed up our metabolism, assist with elimination, and increase the secretion of gastric juices and enzymes.

Remember that cerebral spinal fluid gets balanced by secretion through the nasal sinuses. This activates the nervous system and brings balance to this system.

Lastly, the nervous system and the glandular system work together to modify the chemistry of the brain. The hypothalamus is the go-between for these systems.

Maintaining healthy posture requires a lifelong commitment to your relationship with your breath and all of your senses. Transforming your posture may involve making adjustments in your relationships with others and your perception of the "I" within you.

When you learn how to breathe correctly and connect with the inner being within you, the quality of your daily life changes and so does the expression of your well-being. You become happy and grateful and are able to overcome any challenge or obstacle in your life. Your mind is clearer and you have the ability to reach out and help others.

Body awareness helps you to remember that life is experienced through your body. Treat your body as an "I" instead of an "It". Becoming more aware with greater perception is the key to dissolving all of the negative thoughts and self-talk you may have created throughout your life. Give up blame, fears, the past, judgment, self-criticism, control, attachment, and limiting behaviors (Norton, C, 2013).

Yes, healing your posture is the key to self-discovery. Remember to focus on the diaphragm, pelvic floor region, and transversus abdominus when it comes to movement and exercise. Move from the navel point, relax your eyes, drop your jaw, and breathe in and out of your nose. Stay aware of your body and breathe while you are working out. Don't forget that everything connects within your body and every system works together for optimal performance.

Dig deep for the cause of any problem before making an assumption or judgment and don't forget to be creative. Don't constrict your visual field and keep your eyes wide open to experience every precious moment of life.

Are you transformed? Are you free?

Breathe in life!

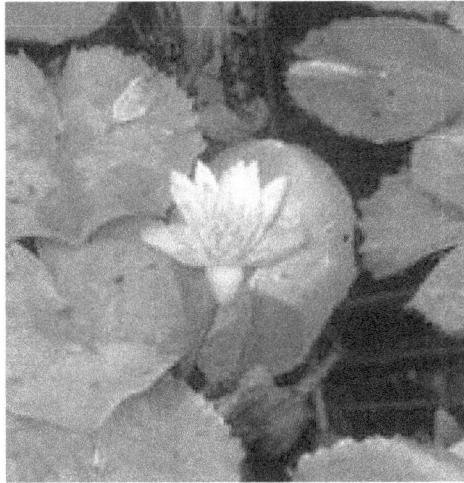

About The Author

MICHELLE LINDSEY-WEHNER's educational preparation and certification includes a Bachelor of Science degree in Kinesiology at Indiana University; a Bachelor of Science degree in Physical Therapy at The Finch University of Health Sciences, Chicago Medical School, now known as Rosalind Franklin University; and a Master of Business Administration in Health Care Management at the University of Phoenix. She is also a Certified Personal Trainer (CPT), KRI Yoga Instructor, a Level 3 Reiki Practitioner, and is certified in Tai massage and Dry Needling. She is currently working on her Doctorate in Physical Therapy from Rosalind Franklin University.

She is a licensed Physical Therapist in three states (Illinois, Arizona, and Colorado) and has over 16 years of experience. A member of the American Physical Therapy Association (APTA) as well its Arizona Chapter, she owns Rising Star Therapy Specialists, LLC, in Phoenix where she specializes in treating pediatric and adult special needs clients.

Throughout her career, Ms. Lindsey has worked as a therapist in various settings, including orthopedics, skilled nursing services, home health, outpatient, and acute care. She has been a guest speaker at the National Spinal Cord Injury Association Conference, the American Physical Therapy Association, the American Recreational Therapy Association, and was the keynote speaker for Rehab Summit in 2009, 2010, and in 2013. She has delivered numerous in-service trainings to schools, day programs, group homes, and state-operated agencies on physical therapy and exercise for persons with disabilities.

She has won national recognition in many areas of fitness. She was a competitive gold medal figure skater, an elite marathon runner on the 1997 United States Maccabiah Open Track and Field Team, a triathlete, and a professional speed skater.

Ms. Lindsey views her clients as unique individuals with varied skills and abilities. She inspires them to extend beyond their best efforts by providing a comfortable, compassionate and respectful environment in which they thrive. Currently, Michelle travels across the United States speaking on three seminar topics:

- Integrating Neurotherapeutic and Sensory Techniques into Therapy for the Special Needs Client;

- A Systems Model Approach to Improving Function, Posture and Scoliosis -- Flexibility and Function;
- Yoga Therapy: Achieving Greater Awareness and Understanding for Healing Our Clients and Ourselves.

Her first book, *The Wellness Equation*, offers hands-on-postures and exercises that promote healing at the crossroads of modern medicine and traditional yoga. *The Metamorphic Gift: Easy, Simple Techniques to Transform Your Life* is a great book for self-healing that integrates the body with breathing and postural exercises using understandable anatomy and physiology.

For more information, please visit: www.risingstartherapyspecialists.com

Bibliography

Allardice, P. (1997). *The art of aromatherapy*. New Jersey: Crescent Books.

Aljasir, B, Bryson, M. & Al-shehri, B. Yoga practice of type II diabetes mellitus in adults: a systematic review. [Abstract] *Evidence-based Complementary and Alternative Medicine* (2008): 1-10.

Amen, D.G. (1999). *Change your brain, change your life: The breakthrough program for conquering anxiety, depression, obsessiveness, anger, and impulsiveness.* New York, NY: Three Rivers.

Ansar Group, Inc. (2014). *Ansar.* Retrieved at http://www.ans-hrv.com/faq.htm.

Answers.com. Transversus abdominis muscle. Available at http://www.answers.com/topic/transversus-abdominis-muscle.

Arambula, P., Peper, E., Kawakami, M. & Gibray, K.H. (2001). The physiological correlates of Kundalni Yoga meditation: A study of a yoga master. *Applied Psychophysiology and Biofeedback,* 26 (2), 147-53.

Acutonics. Use and application of tuning forks. [Article] Available at http://www.acutonics.com/tuning-forks-use.php.

Bagus, J. (2013). Yoga breathing (Pranayan): The importance of breathing. [Article] Available at http://www.abc-of-yoga.com/info/article-printer-version.asp?id=145.

Ballard, K. (2012, Sept.). Laugh your way to better health. *AZnetnews*, 26(4).

Beck, S. (2003). *The teacher's pet*. Crestone, CO: Sue Enterprises.

Behake, E. (1988), Matching. *Somatics,* 18-19.

Bennett, S. & Bennett, R. (2003*). 365 outdoor activities you can do with your child.* Holbrook, MA: Adams Media.

Berg. M., Miles, P., Lee, F. & Lamport, R. (2010). Reiki treatment helps heart attack patients, *Journal of the American College of Cardiology, 56,* 995-996.

Better Day Yoga. Hand mudra. Available at http://betterdayyoga.com/home/mudra-for-powerful-energy/277

Bhajan, Y. (2006). *Kundalini Yoga for youth and joy.* 2nd ed. Santa Cruz, NM: Kundalini Research Institute.

Bhajan, Y. Prana, Vayus, Nadis and Kundalini [lecture transcribed]. 1/1/1976. Yogi Bhajan Lecture Archive. Available at http://fateh.sikhnet.com/sikhnet/articles.nsf/e6a281b4262b05de87256671004e06c5/5e3ca0e44681b b28872576fd007d1744!OpenDocument.

Bhajan, Y. (2007). *The Aquarian teacher level one instructor textbook.* 4th ed. Santa Cruz, NM: Kundalini Research Institute.

Bhajan, Y. (2000). *The master's touch: On being a sacred teacher for the new age.* Revised 1st ed. Santa Cruz, NM: Kundalini Research Institute.

Bharati, S.J. Traditional yoga and meditation of the Himalayan masters: Breathing practices and Pranayama in yoga. [Article] Available at http://swamij.com/breath.htm.

Biology of Kundalini. Neuroendocrine theory of aging. [Article] Available at http://biologyofKundalini.com/article.php?story=NeuroendocrineTheoryofAging

Birdee, G.S., Yeh, G., Wayne, P., Phillips, R., Davis, R. & Gardineo, P. Clinical applications of yoga for the pediatric population: A systematic review. (Abstract) *Academic Pediatrics* 9 (4), 212 – 220. 2009. Available at http://www.ncbi.nlm.nih.gov/pubmed/19608122.

Bond, M. (2007). *The New Rules of Posture.* Rochester, VT: Healing Press.

Bonde, E., Anderson E., Brisman J, Eklof, M., Ringsberg, K.C. & Toren, K. (2012). Dissociation of dysfunctional breathing and odour intolerance among adults in a general-population study. *Clinical Respiratory Journal.*

Boyle, M. Perform better. Are you doing your abdominal training wrong? [Article] Available at http://www.performbetter.com/webapp/wcs/stores/servlet/PBOnePieceView?storeId=10151&catalogId=1075 1&languageId=-1&pagename=79.

Bronfort, G., Maiers, M. J., Evans, R.L., Schulz, C.A., Bracha, Y., Svendsen, K. H., Grimm, R., H. Jr, Owens, E., F. Jr., Garvey, T. A. & Transfeldt, E. E. (2011). Supervised exercise, spinal manipulation and home exercise for chronic low back pain: A randomized clinical trial. *Spine Journal,* 11(7): 585-98.

Brown, J. (1995). *Live and learn and pass it on.* Tennessee: Rutledge Hill Press,

Brown, R. P. and Gerbarg, P. L. (2009). Yoga breathing, meditation, and longevity. *Annals of the New York Academy of Sciences*, 1172, p. 54-62.

Bullen, D. (2012). Yoga for athletic injuries: Personalized poses have a place in rehab. *Advance for Physical Therapy.* King of Prussia, PA: Merion Matters.

Buddiga, P. & Kaliner, M.A. Medscape Reference. (2011). Vocal cord dysfunction. [Article] Available at http://emedicine.medscape.com/article/137782-view.

Budzynski, T. Stanford University. The clinical guide to sound and light. [Article] Available at http://www.stanford.edu/group/brainwaves/2006/theclinicalguidetosoundandlight.pdf.

Bumgardner, W. (2008). How to breathe: Breathing and walking. [Article]. Available at http://walking.about.com/od/fitness/a/breathing.htm.

Byers, D. (1993). *Better health with foot reflexology: The original Ingham Method.* Florida: Ingham Publishing, Inc.

Canadian Lung Association. (2014). COPD [Article] Retrieved at http://www.lung.ca/diseases-maladies/copd-mpoc/breathing-rerspiration

Carey, D. & Franklin, E. (2003). The great elixir: Sound healing, oriental medicine and the three treasures. *California Journal of Oriental Medicine,* 14(2). P. 20-21.

Carey, D. & Muynck, M. Acutonics®: (2002). *There's no place like Ohm: Sound healing, oriental medicine and the cosmic mysteries.* Ilano, NM: Devano Press.

Carey, T. (2011). Comparative effectiveness studies in chronic low back pain: Comment on a randomized trial comparing yoga, stretching, and a self-care book for chronic low back pain. *Archives of Internal Medicine,* DOI: 10.1001/archinternmed.2011.519.

Carpenter, S. (2011). Body of thought: Fleeting sensations and body movements hold away over what we feel and how we think. *Scientific American Mind,* 38-45.

Case-Lo, C. (2012). IBS and serotonin: The brain and stomach link. *Healthline Networks, INC.*

Chaikin, L. (2013, April 19). Vision screening and vision rehab therapy. PESI Seminars. Lecture conducted from Phoenix, AZ.

Chuang, L.H., Soares, M.O., Tilbrook, H., Cox, H., Hewitt, C. E., Aplin, J., Semlyen, A., Trewhela, A., Watt, I. & Torgerson, D. J. (August 2012). A pragmatic multi-centered randomized controlled trial of yoga for chronic low back pain: Economic evaluation. *Spine Journal,* (15).

Cohen, B. B. (2012*). Sensing, feeling, and action.* Ontario: Contact Editions.

Consumer Energy Center (2014). Can lamps cause epileptic or other types of seizures? [Article] Retrieved at http:// eneoia.com/myths/lamps_seizures.html.

Crystalinks. Third eye – pineal gland. Available at http://www.crystalinks.com/thirdeyepineal.html.

Cystic Fibrosis Foundation. (2014). Airway clearance techniques. Retrieved at http://www.cff.org/treatments/therapies/respiratory/airwaysclearence/.

Dale, C. (2009). The Subtle Body: An Encyclopedia of Your Genetic Anatomy. Boulder, CO: Sounds True.

Department of Neurobiology and Developmental Sciences. (2009). Muscles organized by region. University of Arkansas for Medical Sciences.

Department of Nursing. (2013). Health facts for your chest physical therapy.

University of Wisconsin. *Hospitals and Clinics Authority*. p. 1-4.

Deuterman, D. North Carolina Personal Injury Law Advocate. (2010). Alternative health series. Yoga useful for stress release, exercise and pain management. NC: Deuterman Law Group. [Article] Available at http://blog.deutermanlaw.com/workers-compensation-cases/resources-for-injured-workers/pain-management/alternative-health-series-yoga-useful-for-stress-release-exercise-and-pain-management/

Diagram Group. (1983*). The Brain: A User's Manual.* New York, NY: Berkeley Books, 1983.

Doman, G. (1994). *What to do about your brain-injured child._*New York:Avery Publishing Group.

Downing, J. (2008). Light therapy for children and youth. [Article] Sebastopol, CA: Light Therapy Institute. [Article] Available at http://www.growingupeasier.org/index.php?main_page=page&id=159&chapter=3

Dragon bone (long gu). [Article] Retrieved from http://www.acupuncturetoday.com/herbcentral/dragonbone.php.

Dusek, J. A., Oto, H. H., Wohlhueter, A.L., Bhasin, M., Zerbini, L. F., Joseph, M. G., Berson, H. & Libermann, T. A. Genomic counter: Stress changes induced by the relaxation response. [Article] Available at http://www.plosone.org/article/info:doi%2F10.1371%2Fjournal.pone.0002576.

Earls, J. Anatomy Trans: Myofascial Meridians Workshop. Stanley Rosenberg Institute. U.K. [Article] Retrieved on April 15, 2013 from www.Stanleyrosenberg.com.

Ebnezar, J, Nagarathna, R., Yogitha, B. & Nagendra, H. R. (2012). Effect of integrated yoga therapy on pain, morning stiffness and anxiety in OA of the knee joint: A randomized control study. *International Journal of Yoga, 5*:1, 28-36.

Elliot, C. Associate Director, Payment Policy and Advocacy, American Physical Therapy Association and CPT 2010. Current procedural terminology by the American Medical Association.

England, P. Birthing from within class. Phoenix, AZ; June 2011. Details available at http://www.birthingfromwithin.com/.

Engles, L. (2006). Nasal breathing. *District's Ultimate Health and Company*, p.1-5.

Epler, M. & Palmer, L. (1990). *Clinical assessment procedures in physical therapy.* Philadelphia: JB Lippincott.

Exeter Natural Health and Personal Development Blog. (2010). Muscles of the TMJ-jaw pain and headaches. [Article] Retrieved at https:// henrytang.wordpress.com/page/2/

Farabee, M. J. The respiratory system. (2001). Maricopa, AZ: Estrella Mountain Community College, 2001. Article] Available at http://www.emc.maricopa.edu/faculty/farabee/biobk/biobookrespsys.html_.

Ferreti, A., Griffin, K. & Wroth, C. (2012). On your mat . . . get set … GO! *Yoga Journal.* [Article] Retrieved on April 15, 2013, from http://www.yogajournal.com/lifestyle/3162.

Flowers Beauty. Available at http://www.flowersbeauty.info/category.flowers/page/2.

Fortin, M. & Macedo, L. (2013). Multitidus and paraspinal muscle group cross-sectional areas of patients with low back pain and control patients: A systematic review with a focus on blinding. *Physical Therapy Journal*, 93, (7). 873-888.

Foster, M. A. Body-based psychotherapy. *Somatic Patterning*, p. 45-57.

Fren, R. (2012, May). 7 breathing exercises to control asthma. *Health Central,* p.1-9.

Franklin, E., Lamprecht, A. & Juris, B. Vibrational healing: The power of sound to heal. *Light of Consciousness*, 21-22.

Gach, M. (1990). *Accupressure's potent points:A guide to self-care for common ailments.* New York: Bantam Books.

Gallagher, A. (2015). The myofascial component of facial pain. [Article] Retrieved at http://www.pain-education.com/facial-pain.html.

Galantino, M. L., Galbavy, R. & Quinn, L. (2008). *Therapeutic effects of yoga for children: A systematic review of the literature.* Pomona, NJ: Richard Stockton College of New Jersey.

Gardner, A. (2009, June). Yoga helps those with Autism. *Health*, p. 1-2.

Garabedian, H. (2004). *Itsy bitsy yoga.* New York, NY: Fireside.

Generic Look. Autonomic nervous system. [Article] Available at http://genericlook.com/anatomy/Autonomic-Nervous-System.

Gershon, M.D. (1998). *The second brain.* New York, NY: Quill.

Ghiya, S. & Lee, M. (2012). Influence of alternative nostril breathing on heart rate variability in non-practitioners of yogic breathing. *International Journal of Yoga*, 5 (1), 66-69.

Goldstein, S. (2009). Posture: Alternatives to the prevailing paradigm. [Article] Available at http://www.docstoc.com/docs/21154263/Posture--alternatives-to-the-prevailing-paradigm.

Gottlieb, R., Wallace, L.(2001). Syntopic phototherapy. *Journal of Behavioral Optometry.* 12: 2. P. 31. Available at http://www.oepf.org/jbo/journals/12-2%20GottliebWallace.pdf.

Grammatopoulou, E. P., Skordillis, E. K., Stavrou, N., Myrianthefs, P., Karteollotis, K., Baltopoulos, G. & Koutsouki, D. (2011). The effect of physiotherapy-based breathing retraining on asthma control. *Journal of Asthma*, 48:6.

Grles, L. (2006). NASAL breathing. *District's Ultimate Health and Company*, p. 1-5.

Goodman, C. & Snyder, T. (1990). *Differential diagnosis in PT.* Philadelphia, PA: WB Sanders Company.

Group Health Research Institute (2011, October 24). Yoga eases back pain in largest U.S. yoga study to date. *Science Daily.* [Article] Retrieved from http://www.sciencedaily.com/ releases/2011/10/111024164708.htm

Haaz, S. & Bartlett, S. J. (2011). Yoga for arthritis; a scoping review. *Rheum Dis Clin North Am.*, 37(1):33-46.

Hagenan, W. (2010). Yoga for MS patients. *Chicago Tribune.* p. 25.

Hagman, C., Janson, C. & Emtner, M. (2008). A comparison between patients with dysfunctional breathing and patients with asthma. *The Clinical Respiratory Journal,* 2(2), p. 86-91.

Hagman, C., Janson, C., & Emtner, M. (2011). Breathing retraining - A five year follow-up of patients with dysfunctional breathing. *Respiratory Medicine*, 105(8), pg. 1153-9.

Hatfield, F. (2005). *Fitness: The complete guide.* Carpinteria, CA: International Sports Science Association.

Hay, L. (1982). *Heal your body.* Carson, CA: Hay House.

Heasley, S. (2012). Yoga may improve behaviors in kids with autism. *Disability Scoop.* [Article] Retrieved from http://www.disabilityscoop.com

Hendricks, G. (1995). *Conscious breathing.* New York., NY: Bantam.

Hey, L. (2007). Healthy focus community education series. [Article] Raleigh, NC: Duke Raleigh Hospital.

Horan, P.(1992). *Empowerment through Reiki: The path of personal and global transformation.* Twin Lakes, WI: Lotus Light.

Home, N. (2014). Aromatherapy. *NYU Langone Medical Center.* [Article] Retrieved from www.med.nyu.edu/content? Chunk /D=37427.

Hyman, M., Liponis, M. (2005). *Ultraprevention: The 6-week plan that will make you healthy for life.* New York, NY: Atria.

India Parenting. Sarvangasana. [Article] 1999. Available at http://www.indiaparenting.com/alternative-healing/12_760/sarvangasana.html.

Irlen. Home page. Long Beach, CA: Irlen Institute International Headquarters; c1998-12. Available at http://irlen.com/.

Isbit, J. Health benefits of the natural squatting position. [Article] Available at http://naturesplatform.com/health_benefits.html.

Jacques, E. (2010). What is ultrasound therapy? [Article]. Available at http://pain.about.com/od/treatment/f/ultrasound_therapy.htm.
Jarmey, C, Myers, T. (2006). An introduction to the anatomy trains myofascial meridians. Article] In *The concise book of the moving body.* Berkeley, CA: North Atlantic Books.

Jayasinghe, S.R. (2004). Yoga in cardiac health [review]. *European Journal of Cardiovascular Prevention and Rehabilitation* (11) : 369-375. Continuum Heart Institute, Beth Israel Medical Center, NY.

Jennings, J. (2008). Touting tummy time: Infants benefit from early use of position. *Advance for Physical Therapy and Rehab Medicine.* Available at http://physical-therapy.advanceweb.com/Article/Touting-Tummy-Time.aspx.

Jones, M. (2012). Yoga, deep breathing used to address soldier's post-traumatic stress. *Journal Sentinel.* [Article] Retrieved from http://printthis.clickability.com/pt/cpt?expire=7&title=Yoga=de.

Jones, O. (2014). Muscles of mastication [Article] Retrieved at http:// teacmeanatomy.info/head/muscles/mastication/

Jora, J. (1991). *Foot reflexology: A visual guide for self-treatment.* New York, NY: St. Martin's Press.

Kate, Wellness MAMA. (2013). Natural first aid and illness kit. [Article] Retrieved from http://welhersmama.com/3516/natural-first-aid-kit/

Keville, K. (2014). Wellness. *Discovery Fitness & Health.*

Kandoff, L. (2007). *Yoga anatomy.* Champaign, IL: Human Kinetics.

Kaplan, M. (2006). *Seeing through new eyes.* Philadelphia, PA: Jessica Kingsley Publishers.

Keane, S. (2005). *Pilates for core strength: A step-by-step guide to improve core strength and stability.* Jackson, TN: Main Street Publishing.

Keller, E. (1991). *The complete home guide to aromatherapy.* H J Kramer, Tiburon, CA.

Kepner, J.I. (1993). *Body process: Working with the body in psychotherapy.* San Francisco, CA: Jossey-Bass, Inc.

Kim, Wook, Lee, Sang-Ho, Lee, Dong Yeob. (2011). Changes in the cross-sectional area of multifidus and psoas in unilateral sciatica caused by lumbar disc hemiation. *Journal of Korean Neurosurgical Society.* 50:201-204.

Khalsa, D.S., Anen, D., Hanks, C., Money, N., Newberg, A. (2009). Cerebral blood flow changes during chanting meditation. *Nuclear Medicine Communications.* [Article] 1-Available at http://www.alzheimersprevention.org/JrnlofNucMedComms0909.pdf.

Khalsa, D. S. & Stauth, C. (2001). *Meditation as Medicine.* New York, NY: Atria.

Khalsa, D.S. DrDharma.com. "Kirtan Kriya." Page. [Article] Available at http://drdharma.com/utility/showArticle/?objectID=249.

Khalsa, M. K. (2008). *Meditation for addictive behavior: A system of yogic science with nutritional formulas.* (2nd ed.) Minneapolis, MN: Itasca Books.

Khalsa, M.K. (2010). Yoga therapy today: Manage the future with grace. *SuperHealth.* [Article] Available at http://super-health.net/articles-and-press/yoga-therapy-today-article/.

Khalsa, N.S. (2010). *The art, science, and application of Kundalini yoga.* (3rd ed.) Dubuque, IA: Kendall Hunt.

Khalsa, S.K. (1998). *Fly like a butterfly. 1st ed.* Portland, OR: Rudra Press.

Khalsa, S.P.K. (1996). *Kundalini yoga: The flow of eternal power.* CA: Berkeley Publishing Group.

Khalsa, S.S., Rudrauf, D., Damasio, A.R., Davidson, R.J., Lutz, A., Tranel, D. (2008) Interoceptive awareness in experienced meditators. *Psychophysiology* 45: 671-677.

Khalsa, S.S.K. (2010). When did yoga therapy become a 'field'? *International Journal of Yoga Therapy.*

Khalsa, T.T.K. (2007). *Conscious pregnancy: The gift of giving life.* Espanola, NM: 3HO Women.

Kliger, B., Lynton, H. & Shiflett, S. (2002). Yoga in stroke rehabilitation: A systematic review and results of a pilot study. In *Top Stroke Rehabilitation.* 14(4), p. 1-8.

Koenig, K.P., Buckley, R. A. & Garg, S. (2012). Efficacy of the get ready to learn yoga program among children with autism spectrum disorders: A pretest-posttest Control group design. *American Journal of Occupational Therapy*, 66 (5), 538-46.

Kolar, P., Sulc, J., Kyncl, M., Sanda, J., Cakrt, O., Andel, R., Kumagai, K. & Kobesova, A. (2012). Postural function of the diaphragm in persons with and without chronic low back pain. *Journal of Orthopaedic and Sports Physical Therapy*, 42(4):352-62.

Kornberg, C. OptusNet. What is scoliosis? [Article.] Available at http://members.optusnet.com.au/physio/scoliosis.html.

Kundalini Research Institute. (2007). .*Kundalini yoga: Sadhana guidelines. (*2nd ed.) Santa Cruz, NM: Kundalini Research Institute.

Kundalini Research Institute. (2010). *Owner's manual for the human body.* (Revised ed.) Santa Cruz, NM: Kundalini Research Institute.

Kundalini Yoga Info Center. Life nerve, sex nerve, mind nerve. [Article] Available at http://www.Kundaliniyogainfocntr.com/page/Life+Nerve,+Sex+Nerve,+Mind+Nerve.

Kupnik, D. (2003). Expert-view Pranayama (breathing exercises) in light of contemporary science. [Article] Retrieved at www.yogaindailylife.org/knowledge/yoga-and-health/expert-v

Lee, D. & Lee, L. J. (2011). *The pelvic girdle: An integration of clinical expertise and research* (4th ed). Edinburgh: Elsevier, Ltd.

Lee, D. (2011). Understand your back and pelvic girdle. [Article] Available at http://dianelee.ca/education/article_understanding_back_pain.php.

Living with cerebral palsy. Dolphin therapy. Available at
http://www.livingwithcerebralpalsy.com/dolphin-cerebral.php.

Lodge, E. (2006). *Primal energetics: Emotional intelligence in action.* Charleston, SC: BookSurge.

Luby, J. L., Barch, D.M., Belden, A., Gaffey, M.S., Tillman, R., Babb, C., Nishino, T., Suzuki, H. & Botteron, K.N. (2012). Maternal support in early childhood predicts larger hippocampal volumes at school age. *Proceedings of the National Academy of Sciences.*

Luby, T. (1998). *Children's book of yoga – Games and exercises mimic plants and animals and objects.* Santa Fe, NM: Clear Light Publishing.

Lung Disease and Respiratory Health Center. Retrieved at
http://www.webmail.com/lung/obstructive-and-restrictive-lung-disease.

MA, Yun-Tao, MA, Mila, and Cho, Zang Hee. (2005). *Biomedical acupuncture for pain management: An integrative approach.* St. Louis, Missouri: Elsevier.

Marriage rescue for omen. Chakra affirmations. Available at
http://www.1lovespirit.com/affirmations-chakras.html.

Mc Ardle, D. & Katch, F. D. (1991). *Exercise Physiology.* (3rd Edition). PA: Lea and Fabiger.

McCarty, R., Bradley, R.T. & Tomasino, D. (2004-2005) Shift at the frontiers of consciousness. *The Resonant Heart.* [Article] Available at http://media.noetic.org/uploads/files/s5_mccraty.pdf.

Michael, A. (2011). Strength training with human kinetics. *Live Strong* [Article] Available at http://www.livestrong.com/article/305190-strength-training-with-human-kinetics/.

Mini color therapy chart. Australia: Dynamo House. See www.alibaba.com

Myers, T. (2006). Early dissective evidence. Anatomy trains, P.16-18. [Article] Available at http://www.anatomytrains.com/uploads/rich_media/ATDiss-1.pdf.

Melina, R. (March 9, 2011). Why is the medical symbol a snake on a stick. Article retrieved at http://www.livescience.com/33104-why-is-the-medical-symbol-a-snake-on-a-stick.html

Naess, I. (2008). *Colour energy for body and soul.* Vancouver, B.C.: Colour Energy Corp.

National Heart, Lung, and Blood Institute. What is COPD? Retrieved at
http://www.nhlbi.gov/health/health-topics/topics/copd/printall...imd....

Natural Ways. Adrenal weakness. Available at http://naturalways.com/adrenal.htm.

Newton, A. C. (1995). Basic concepts in the theory of Hubert Godard. [Article] Rolf Lines, *P.* 33-43 [Article] Available at
http://www.somatics.de/Godard/BasicConcepts.pdf.

Newton, A. C. (1997). Breathing in the Gravity Field. *Rolf Lines.* P. 27-40. [Article] Available at http://www.alinenewton.com/pdf-articles/breathing-article.pdf.

Newton, A. C. (2004). Core stabilization, core coordination. [Article] Available at http://www.alinenewton.com/pdf-articles/core.htm.

Nicholson, D., Examiner. (2010). September is National Yoga Month. [Article] Available at http://www.examiner.com/alternative-medicine-in-detroit/september-is-national-yoga-month.

Nick, K., Nick, V. "How to Grow a Better Brain -- Lobes of the Brain." Available at http://library.thinkquest.org/J002391/functions.html.

Nielsen, M., Keefe, F., Bennell, K. & Jull, G. (2014). Physical therapist -- Delivered cognitive behavioral therapy; A qualitative study of physical therapists' perceptions and experiences. *PT Journal*, 94(2): 197-210.

Nietfeld, EMI. (2012, April). Study: Yoga can improve mental health. *The Harvard Crimson.* [Article} Retrieved from http://www.thrcrimson.com/article/2012/4/12/yoga-mental-health-study/.

Nijs, J., Meeus, M., Cagnie, B., Roussel, N. A., Dolphens, M., Van Oosterwijck, J. & Danneels, L. (2014). A modern neuroscience approach to chronic spinal pain: Combining pain neuroscience educationwith cognition-targeted motor control training. *Physical Therapy*: 2014 May: 94(5): 730-8. doi: 10.2522/ptj.20130258. Epub 2014 Jan 30.

Neuroscience education with cognition-targeted motor control training. *Physical Therapy*, 94(5), 730-738. Accessed February 19, 2016. http://dx.doi.org/10.2522/ptj.20130258

Norton, C. 15 things you should give up to be happy. [Article} Retrieved from www.thoughtcatalog.com.

Novella, S. (2010). Science-based medicine. *National Health Interview Survey 2007 – CAM Use by Adults.* Available at http://www.sciencebasedmedicine.org/?p=203.

Nucleus Medical Media. The Parasympathetic Nervous System – Medical illustration, human anatomy drawing. Kennesaw, GA: Nucleus Medical Media. Available at http://catalog.nucleusinc.com/generateexhibit.php?ID=1885.

O'Donnell, L. (1999). Music and the brain. [Article] Available at http://www.cerebromente.org.br/n15/mente/musica.html.

Ogle, M. About.com. (2010). Anatomy of the spine. [Article] Available at http://pilates.about.com/od/technique/ss/human-spine-anatomy.htm.

Oliver, J. (2014). The muscles of mastication. [Article] Retrieved at http://teachmeanatomy.info/head/muscles/mastication/.

Optimal Breathing. Nose breathing. [Article] Available at http://breathing.com/articles/nose-breathing.htm.

Oregon Optometric Physicians Association Children's Vision Committee.(2000). *Handbook for Educators and Parents on the Effects of Vision on Learning and School Performance.* Milwaukee, OR: Oregon Optometric Physicians Association.

Pearlscott, M. (1999-2015). What is fascia? Retrieved at
http://www.treatmentmassage.com/structural-integration/what-is-fascia.html

Pederson, T. (2012). Classroom yoga improves behaviors of kids with autism. *Psych Central.*
[Article] Retrieved from
http://psychcentral.com/2012/10/15/classroom-yoga-improves-behavior-of-kids-with-
autism/46081.html

Pert, C. (1997). *Molecules of emotion: The science behind mind-body medicine.* New York, NY:
Touchstone.

Phillips, A. Treating causes at cell level. *NeuroLink.* [Article] Available at
http://www.neurolinkglobal.com/T-Cell-level_436.aspx.

Proactive Healthnet. (2001). How light therapy works. [Article] Available at
http://www.proactivehealthnet.com/healthBB/archive/index.php?t-848.html.

Reents, S. (2012). The athlete in m*e*. *Yoga.* [Article] 2012. Available at:
http://www.athleteinme.com/ArticleView.aspx?id=265.

Rose, D. Nose breathing vs. mouth breathing: Nose breathing is optimal. See why and how below.
[Article] Retrieved at www.Breathing.com/articles/nose-breathing.htm.

Rothschild, B. (2000). *The Body Remembers: The Physiology of Training and Trauma Treatment.*
New York, NY: Norton.

Sandalcidi, D. (2011). The pelvic floor: The missing link in pelvic girdle stability. [Article]
Phoenix, AZ: Woman's Health Conference.

Scoliosis Association, Inc. Scoliosis facts. [Article] Available at http://scoliosis-assoc.org/.

Shelton, D.L. (2010). Drug firms pay docs millions *Chicago Tribune.*

Sinclair, J. (2007). The violet flame and sounds of music. [Article] *The Violet Ray.* Alberta, CA:
Red Deer.

Schleip, R. (2003). Fascial Plasticity: A new neurobiological explanation. *Journal of Bodywork and
Movement Therapies. 7* (1):11-19 and 7 (2), 104-116.

Schell, S (2001). The Shenoid bone: A cornerstone of health. Retrieved at
http://www.bodywisdomcst.com/sphenoid-bone-a-cornerstone-of-health.html

Schmid, A.,Van Puymbroeck, M. V., Altenburger, P.,Schalk, N., Dierks, T., Miller, K., Damush, T.,
Bravata, D. & Williams, L. (2012). Poststroke balance improves with yoga: A pilot study. *Stroke,*
43: 2402-2407.

Seattle Community Network (2007). Florescent lighting and other optical issues. Retrieved at
http://www.scn.org/autistics/fluorescents.html

Seekers, J. (2011). Aromatherapy. University of Maryland Medical Center. [Article] Retrieved,
from http://umm.edu/health/medical/altmed/treatment/aromatherapy.

Seikel, J.A., King, D. W. & Drumright, D. G. (2010). *Anatomy and physiology for speech, language, and hearing.* Clifton Park, New York: Delmar.

Shaw, G., (1999), Mozart effect research. *The Journal of Neurological Research.* Retrieved at http://www.angelfire.com/biz/acousticdigest/mozartmind.html

Shreya, G. & Lee, M. (2012). Influence of alternate nostril breathing on heart rate variability in non-practitioners of yogic breathing.*International Journal of Yoga.* (5), 66-69.

Sherman, K. D., Cherkin, D. C., Wellman, R. D., Cook, A. J., Hawkes, R. J., Delaney, K. & Deyo, R. A. (2011). A randomized trial comparing yoga stretching and a self-care book for chronic low back pain. *Archives of Internal Medicine*, DOI: 10.1001/Archinternmed.2011.524.

Smiths, N. (1984). Moving from within. *Naropa Magazine,* p. 7-12.

Sodhi, C., Singh, S. & Dandona, P. K., (2009, April). A study of the effect of yoga training and pulmonary functions in patients with bronchial asthma. *Indian Journal of Physiology and Pharmacology*, 53. (2), pg. 169-74.

Spencer, S. (2009). The art of mastering movement. Multifidus Muscle – the Core: Part 3 – Week 4 of Pilates. Santa Cruz, CA: Pacific Movement Center. [Article] Available at http://www.stephanie-spencer.com/category/the-core/page/2.

Tarpan, F. (1988). *Healing Massage Techniques.* E. Norwich, CT: Appleton & Lange.

The Autism Coach. Gifted and disabled: Intriguing connections between giftedness and autism, music, and language. [Article] Available at http://www.autismcoach.com/Articles.asp?ID=296

The Caroline Theme (2014). What is myofascia and myofascial release? Retrieved at https://vicmassage.com/2014/11/12/what-is-myofascia-and-myofascial-release/

The Learning Curve. (2004*). Brain activation patterns.* Lancaster, PA. Available at http://www.brain-trainer.com/brain_patterns.

Thomas, P. (2004). *Under the weather: How weather and climate affect our health.* London: Fusion.

Thompson, J. D. The clinical use of sound. Carlsbad, CA: Center for Neuroacoustic Research. [Article] Available at http://www.neuroacoustic.com/clinical_services/html.

Toneatto, T. & Nguyen, L. (2007). Does mindfulness meditation improve anxiety and mood symptoms? A review of the controlled research. [Article.] *Canadian Journal of Psychiatry.* 52 (4), 260-266. Ottawa, ONT: Canadian Psychiatric Association.

Tilbrook, H. E., Cox, H., Hewitt, C. E. et al. (2011). Yoga for persistent pain: New findings and directions for an ancient practice. *Pain,* 152(3):477-480.

TMJ and MFR. [Article] Retrieved at www.myofascialrelease.co.uk.

Tribune Media Services. (2010). Yoga could be good for cardiovascular disease. *Chicago Tribune.*

Umphred, D. (1996). An integrated approach to adult neurological deficits with head injured tonal clients. *Pacific Coast Services*: Illinois, 3-5.

Umphred, D. (1990). *Neurological Rehabilitation*. St. Louis: The C.V. Mosby Company.

UMMC. (2014). Lung Disease. *UMMC,* p. 1-3.

University of Maryland Medical Center. Melatonin. (2011). Baltimore, MD: University of Maryland Medical Center, [Article.] Available at http://www.umm.edu/altmed/articles/melatonin-000315.htm.

Valladares, E. Connecting with light. The Chakras. Available at http://connectingwithlight.com/chakra.htm.

Van De Graaff, K. (1989). *Human Anatomy & Physiology Study Cards*. 4th ed. Dubuque, IA: Brown Publishing.

Vázquez-Vandyck, M., Roman, S., Vázquez, J. L., Huacuja, L., Khalsa, G., Troyo-Sanroman, R. & Panduro, A. (2007). Effect of breathwalk on body composition, metabolic and mood state in chronic hepatitis C patients with insulin resistance syndrome. *World Journal of Gastroenterology.* 13_(46): 6213 – 6218. [Article.] Available at http://www.wjgnet.com/1007-9327/13/6213.pdf.

Vemier, (2014). *Human Physiology.* Beaverton, Oregon: Vemier Software and Technology.

Vuenk82. Muscles of respiration. [Article] Retrieved at http://quizlet.com/2899683/muscles_of-respiration-flash-cards/.

Wax, H. (2006). We got the beat. *Science and Theology News.* Available at http://www.wellness-institute.org/images/We Got the Beat Rhythm_affects_the_Brain_-_8-8-2006.pdf.

Wehner, M. L. (2012). *The wellness equation: Exploring the healing connection between yoga and medicine.* Arizona: The Yogacademy.

Wellesley, MA: (2005). Wellesley College Hippocratic Society. Available at http://www.wellesley.edu/Activities/homepage/hippocratic/oath.html.

Wilder, B. (2013). Hiatal hernia: Self-adjustment techniques and treatments. [Article] Retrieved at www.healingnaturallybybee.com/hiatal-hernia-self-adjustment-technique-treatments/

Wikipedia. Available at http://en.wikipedia.org/wiki/Antagonist_%28muscle%29.
Wikipedia. Available at http://en.wikipedia.org/wiki/Circulatory_system.
Wikipedia. Available at http://en.wikipedia.org/wiki/Human_skeleton.
Wikipedia. Available at http://en.wikipedia.org/wiki/Muscles_of_respiration.
Wikipedia. Available at http://en.wikipedia.org/wiki/Osmolarity.
Wikipedia. Available at http://en.wikipedia.org/wiki/Respiratory_system.
Wikipedia. Available at http://en.wikipedia.org/wiki/Diaphragm_%28anatomy%29.
Wikipedia. Available at http://en.wikipedia.org/wiki/Vacuum_exercise.
Wikipedia. Available at http://en.wikipedia.org/wiki/Visual_system.

Why babies breathe more rapidly than adults. [Article] Retrieved at http://somethingnewlearnedeveryday.blogspot.com.br/2010/01/why-babies-breathe-more-rapidly-than.html

Worldly Minds. (2013). Your voice commands your mind, body and spirit. [Article] Retrieved from www. worldly minds.com.

Wren, A. A., Wright, M. A., Carson, J. W. et al. (2011). Yoga for persistent pain: New findings and directions for an ancient practice. *Pain*, 152 (3):477-480.

Zhang, P. (2015) Meditations effects on alpha brain waves: A new study at Brown University. [Article] Retrieved at blog.lumosity.com/meditation/2/Brain, Health/Brain Research, Science.

Zope, S. A. & Zope, R. A., (2013). Sudarshan Kriya Yoga: Breathing for health. *International Journal of Yoga,* 6(1), 4-10.

www.ingramcontent.com/pod-product-compliance
Lightning Source LLC
Chambersburg PA
CBHW080421270326
41929CB00018B/3117